MW00777850

to you...

-R. Wayne Morgan

11-16			
3-22-17			
21-2-17			

Demco, Inc. 38-293

Happy Birthday – You're Old

A Boomer's Guide to Aging
and Other Unexpected Developments

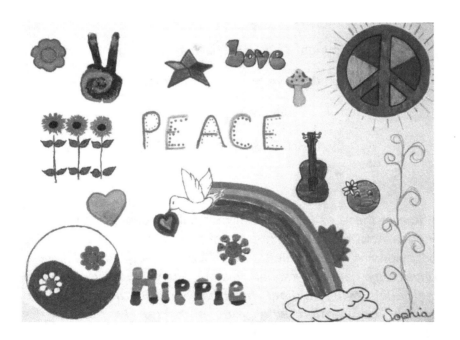

R. Wayne Morgan

Happy Birthday – You're Old

A Boomer's Guide to Aging and Other Unexpected Developments

R. Wayne Morgan

2016 Paperback Edition

Copyright © 2016 by R. Wayne Morgan

Cover Art by Carolyn Grace

ISBN: 978–0–9845048–8–6

Some of these essays contain medical anecdotes and advice. Please note that the author is not a doctor. (He may also be occasionally uninformed or misinformed.) *In addition, physiology and personal history vary greatly between individuals.* **All medical information and health advice should be verified with your physician to confirm its application to your unique situation.**

I welcome comments and suggestions for improvement at the email address below. Thanks.

-R. Wayne Morgan, Publisher
rwaynemorgan@comcast.net

To My Generation

Proceeds from this book go to:

The American Cancer Society – in memory of Melody

The Nature Conservancy – in honor of Carolyn

Contents

Contents

Is This Book For You?

If you are age 9 to 49:

I wrote this book for and about Baby Boomers. It focuses on aging. You may find it irrelevant because old age still seems a long way off. I can only suggest that it is never too early to learn about your body and the health habits that contribute to successful aging.

If you are the child of a Baby Boomer, perhaps you bought this book for your parents. In that case, they are fortunate. This book will help them maintain their health for years to come. You are a good daughter or son.

If you just turned 30, 40, or 50:

You may have received this book as a gag gift. Someone wanted to make a big deal about your age. I put the phrase "You're Old" in the title in hopes of selling a boatload of copies to people who want to rub it in your face.

Keep the book. Re-gift it back to the person the next time *they* have a milestone birthday.

If you are in your 50s or 60s:

You are a Baby Boomer. This book is for you.
— It will provide some understanding of the changes
      you are noticing in your body.
— It will help you avoid or delay some aspects of aging.
— It will provide opportunities to reflect on your life.

If nothing else, it contains some relevant short essays to read while sitting in the bathroom.

What Is In This Book?

We Boomers are now aging. This provides us with a new set of experiences to share. Following our tradition, we will bring our own unique style to this life stage.

Consistent with our natural optimism, terms like "healthy aging" and "successful aging" are attractive to us. We have always wanted to control our own destiny.

Scientists tell us that some of aging is beyond our control—written in our genes. But we are not going down without a fight. To the extent possible, we will be in charge of our aging as no generation before.

Section I of this book is entitled *Body Blows*. These essays introduce common health issues of aging, providing understandable physiological explanations. They highlight features of aging that can be prevented or postponed by healthy lifestyle choices.

I take the liberty to modify a twentieth-century prayer attributed to American theologian Reinhold Niebuhr:

> *God, grant me the serenity to accept the aging I cannot change,*
> *The courage to slow the aging I can,*
> *And the wisdom to know the difference.*

Section II of this book is entitled *Memories and Musings*. These essays are about my experiences as a Baby Boomer. You may relate to some of them, prompting you to reflect on your own life. At our age, a little reflection seems appropriate.

Prologue: Who Are the Boomers?

We are the product of a demographic anomaly. Everyone knows the story: Horny men returned en masse from World War II and happily contributed to the production of millions of babies—about seventy-five million in the United States between 1946 and 1964. This produced a "python swallowing a pig" bulge in the population graph like no other in history. By 1964, 40% of the U.S. population was Boomer—under age nineteen.

The origin of the term "Baby Boomer" is debated, but many credit *New York Post* financial columnist Sylvia Porter. She wrote:

"Take the 3,548,000 babies born in 1950, bundle them into a batch, bounce them all over the bountiful land that is America. What do you get? Boom. The biggest, boomiest boomy boom ever known in history."

The term "Baby Boomer" evolved and we have worn the label ever since.

I've always been a little uncomfortable being grouped together with those that are as much as seventeen years younger. (I was born in 1947.) In our rapidly changing culture, even a few years difference in age can impact a life with an entirely new set of circumstances. For example, my high school graduation yearbook of 1965 looks very similar to those from the 1950s—boys have short haircuts; girls have long skirts. The focus is on cheerleaders, clubs, sports, and the prom queen.

Three years later—when my brother graduated—boys have long hair, girls have short skirts, and the entire yearbook is a protest of the Vietnam War.

During my high school years, the most daring of my friends might sneak a beer into a Saturday night party. For my brother's friends, marijuana use was common—and some were experimenting with LSD, amphetamines, and other drugs. Same neighborhood, same school, but an entirely different set of experiences.

Broadening the time frame, coming of age during the reign of the Beatles and British Invasion was very different than coming of age to the soundtrack of the Bee Gees' *Saturday Night Fever*. Certainly, growing up in an affluent California suburb provided me with different experiences than Boomers who grew up in the urban ghettos of Harlem or East LA. Of course, the process of being drafted and sent to war in Vietnam profoundly affected some Boomers.

We do well to remember that all generalizations are lies—even this one. Despite being lumped together with the demographers' alliterative label, we are a diverse generation.

Can we say anything meaningful about Baby Boomers as a whole? In an attempt to add precision to his commentary, Steve Gillon (*Boomer Nation*) distinguishes between the Early Boomers (born 1946-1957) and Late Boomers (1958-1964):

> "The early generation of Baby Boomers grew up with rock and roll, the Mickey Mouse Club, prosperity, crew cuts, the idealism of John F. Kennedy, and the social struggles of the 1960s. A child born in 1964 confronted a world of oil embargos, stagflation, Watergate, sideburns, and disco balls."

Gillon suggests that Early Boomers spent much of their lives trying to reconcile their youthful idealism with social reality, while Late Boomers had less idealism to compromise.

Early Boomers have been described as experimental, free spirited, social cause oriented, and quick to reject traditional values. The overriding influence in their lives was the affluence of post-war America in the 1950s. We are more likely to have a genuine expectation that the world (and individuals) will improve with time.

Late Boomers were less optimistic and more cynical. The Vietnam War, the Cold War, Watergate, Nixon's resignation, raging inflation, and the loss of 1950's innocence dominated the culture of their childhood.

I will be writing from the perspective of an Early Boomer. Despite our broad spectrum of individual differences, I have always felt a kinship with others born in the late 1940s and early 1950s. Many of us shared a carefree, affluent, suburban childhood (as exaggerated in the movie *Pleasantville*). Some have argued that this gave us a feeling of entitlement. I prefer to see this as the foundation for our prevailing sense of optimism.

The turbulent zeitgeist of the 1960s also forged our Early Boomer identity. To the soundtrack of protest folk music that evolved into electrified rock and roll, we bonded as a group and separated ourselves from the prevailing culture as no previous generation. When I am with other Early Boomers, there is a shared knowing, a mutual understanding, an unspoken bond of common experience.

I never served in the military, yet I feel a sincere empathy for those in my generation who were drafted to fight in Vietnam. Contrasting the images on the nightly news at the time with the pronouncements of government leaders, I learned to question authority and seek my own truth.

I never danced in the mud of Max Yasgur's farm or walked the streets of Haight-Ashbury with a flower in my hair, yet I appreciate the need to break the bonds of traditional culture and take a stand for personal freedom. I learned to respect the right of each person to follow her or his own path.

I never burned my Draft Card or lay down in front of a military transport train, yet I learned to support political change by becoming informed, expressing my opinion—and voting.

I never attended a feminist protest rally or marched in the South for racial justice, but I worked to overcome my stereotypes and learned to treat others with acceptance and respect.

Like so many of our generation, I have been a quiet revolutionary. I am proud to be a Boomer.

Introduction

So why do we have to age, anyway? It is little comfort to say, "It is the nature of things." That is, however, the truth. Nature has programmed us—and all other living things—to age and die. It is literally in our DNA. It would take a class in evolutionary biology to fully explain, but let me attempt a short version here.

When life arose on Earth, it had to deal with a planet that is constantly changing. Lakes become forests. Forests become deserts. Deserts rise up to become mountains. Mountains erode into the sea. Storms, droughts, heat waves, ice ages, earthquakes, volcanoes—in the big picture of geologic time, precious life has always been living on the edge of destruction. And of course, all forms of life are constantly threatened by other species competing for the same resources.

For life forms to survive on a changing, unpredictable, and competitive planet, DNA had to be able to change and adapt. In other words, the book of life had to be easily edited. Nature created the process of evolution to provide the most chances for life to succeed.

Through the magic of mutations (that produce new genes) and sexual reproduction (that produces new combinations of genes), every generation of a species contains individuals with a wide range of traits. Some of these trait combinations will be successful—lead to survival and reproduction—and other combinations will not.

Evolution requires each generation to get out of the way so the next generation can try new gene combinations—new chances to adapt to a changing environment. Thus, our DNA is programmed for aging and death.

At this point, scientists do not understand all of the genetic instructions that produce aging. One thing they have observed is that the cells of each species seem to have limits on their ability to reproduce. Lab mice live an average of three years, with their cells able to divide about 15 times before they degrade and die. Galapagos turtles may live two hundred years, with their cells programmed to divide as many as 110 times. Maximum human lifespan is considered to be about one hundred twenty years, with each of our cells dividing an average of about 50 times.

As our cells lose the ability to produce healthy young replacements by cell division, our body accumulates damage and degrades. We call this aging.

The harsh reality is that nature does not care about our survival as individuals. It only cares about the survival of our species—specifically, the survival of the DNA that produces our species.

Future generations are likely to have options for life extension that now exist only in science fiction. For us, aging and death are the facts of life. The best we can do as individuals is to maximize our health while accepting the inevitability of our death. Mother Nature will ultimately insist that we Boomers leave the stage.

Before I cease my strutting and fretting (remember your Shakespeare?), I decided to write a book about healthy aging and being a Baby Boomer. Why?

I am writing this book because I enjoy writing.

I am writing this book because I like to reflect.

I am writing this book because I want to help others.

I am writing this book *now* because the timing is right. This year (2016) the oldest Boomers turn seventy. That is a mind-boggling milestone. Already the youngest Boomers have passed the age of fifty. Even for a generation that tends toward denial, these developments come as a shock.

"Don't trust anyone over thirty." Jack Weinberg spoke these words during the 1965 Free Speech Movement at UC Berkeley. This admonition became emblematic of our rejection of the cultural norms of previous generations.

"Don't trust anyone over eighty?" Somehow, half a century later, our youthful mantra loses its rebellious bravado. Aging and dying will fade our identity and erase our historic exceptionality. We are, after all, just a footnote in the larger human saga.

But let's not get depressed. We are not dead yet. In fact, we have a lot of living left to do. We have the luxury of savoring our past while living to the fullest in the present. As John Denver sang, "It turns me on to think of growing old."

Let's remember that we Boomers have always supported each other and found strength in numbers—our most defining characteristic. If we maintain our health and energy, we can continue to shape our culture in positive ways, working toward a better world for our grandchildren.

We can continue to expand our legacy.

As we came of age, some of us marched in formation before heading to Vietnam. Some of us marched carrying signs to protest social injustice. Most of us did not march at all—except perhaps to our local record store to get the latest album by the Beatles, Stones, or Dylan. (*More of the Monkeys* was the top selling album of 1967. Anyone willing to admit to buying it?)

Since those formative years, we have all walked our individual life path with its ups, downs, and unexpected turns. Now, in this final leg of our remarkable journey, perhaps there is comfort in knowing that we all walk arm in arm.

The following pages will include some personal experiences, some intellectual preparation, and some nostalgic reflection.

Enjoy.

-- *Wayne*

"If I'd known I was going to live this long,
I'd have taken better care of myself."

–Eubie Blake before a ragtime piano performance at age 99.

Section I

Body Blows

Note: The issues of aging discussed in *Section I* represent a small sampling of the hundreds that might be relevant to any particular individual. In addition, each brief essay is only an introduction to the topic. It is my hope that you will follow up with your own research to be fully informed. Please consult an appropriate health care professional regarding any question of concern.

****

Passages in the essays included below this line are intended for readers who desire an extended, sometimes more technical discussion of the topic.

A Game of Takeaway # 1

When my father was in his late seventies, I picked him up from his assisted living residence to go out to lunch. At the restaurant, he ordered a bowl of soup to start. I watched with some discomfort as he fumbled with a package of saltine crackers the server had provided. Try as he might, he could not tear the thin cellophane wrapper—and each attempt crushed the crackers into smaller crumbs.

With the tension rising for both of us, I finally intervened. "May I help you?" I was concerned that my question might anger him. Instead, his face expressed relief. "Sure, my hands are just not strong enough anymore." That was one of my first introductions to the joys of aging.

Physiologists tell us that we lose as much as 1% of our muscle mass each year as we age. The process begins subtly after age thirty and accelerates after age sixty-five. Like so much of the aging process, it is a game of takeaway.

I have no trouble believing that I am significantly weaker than I was as a young man. After all, I used to dunk a basketball with a vertical leap of over thirty inches (not great by NBA standards, but respectable for a skinny college bench player). Now my best jump would be much less than twenty inches. I could measure it precisely—but I am afraid I would hurt myself.

For we who are males, self-image and self-esteem intertwine with our muscle strength. When my wife hands me a jar and asks me to open it, my masculinity is on the line.

So far, I have usually met the challenge, but I know my days as a silverback gorilla are numbered. I will invest in lid opening tools. The principle of leverage will save my manhood for a while longer.

The effects of muscle loss go well beyond everyday frustrations like opening a jar—or package of crackers. Loss of strength is a primary contributing factor to falls in the elderly. (Reduced balance skills also contribute.) Two and a half *million* older Americans are treated in emergency rooms for falls each year. Seven hundred thousand are hospitalized for severe injuries ranging from head trauma to hip fractures. Twenty-five thousand die.

In these writings, I want to focus on the positive. Consider that two-thirds of all Americans over the age of sixty-five manage to avoid falling each year! And that number could be much higher if older people realized the value of strength training.

Research has shown that individuals who maintain a typical American activity level (labeled semi-sedentary) lose an average of 6% of muscle mass per decade after age twenty—or 30% total by age seventy. By contrast, *those that are physically active with appropriate strength training may lose only 2% per decade—or 10% by age seventy.*

Maintaining our muscle function for as long as possible is one of the most important anti-aging steps we can take. Keeping our legs strong and flexible helps prevent falls. Preserving upper body strength enhances our self-sufficiency and allows us to continue with activities that bring us joy and satisfaction.

14

For these reasons, the smartest of my friends have joined a gym, hired a personal trainer, begun yoga classes, or (at least) walk regularly. I am not Mr. Fitness, but I try to do some kind of physical activity for 30 or more minutes every day. (On days when I don't play pickleball, I use an exercise bike, lift weights, or take an extended walk.)

Muscle strength is just one of the takeaways of aging. In fact, aging is defined by the takeaways. Skin tone, vision, hearing, hair color, flexibility, sex drive, short-term memory—and the list goes on. Section I essays focus on some physical and mental health takeaways of aging and choices we can make to go down fighting.

****

As we age, both muscle mass and muscle strength decrease. The process is called *sarcopenia*. Several factors are at work, including:

- Cells responsible for muscle regeneration (satellite cells) are produced in smaller numbers as we age.
- Hormone levels that support muscle growth (growth hormone, testosterone, insulin-like growth factor) decline.
- Protein synthesis within muscle tissue slows.
- The number of mitochondria (cell energy organelles) within muscle cells decreases.
- The number of motor neurons (nerve cells) declines, leading to atrophy of muscle fibers that are no longer stimulated.

One logical strategy to reduce muscle loss would seem to be supplementation of the hormones that stimulate muscle growth. Unfortunately, studies have not consistently shown improved muscle strength with hormone supplementation—while worrisome side effects have been shown. For example, testosterone may increase the risk of blood clots and prostate cancer. Human growth hormone may produce fluid retention, diabetes, and speed tumor growth.

At this point, regular exercise and strength training are the most effective ways to prevent loss of muscle mass with aging. A complete program would include:

Endurance Exercise Low-impact aerobic exercises (walking, cycling, swimming, dancing, etc.) are recommended for both muscle tone and cardiovascular health. *Walking two miles a day may reduce mortality rates by 50%.*

Resistance Exercise The consensus today is that resistance exercise (free weights, exercise machines) should be performed at least twice each week. Professional guidance is recommended to start in order to avoid injury and maximize benefits.

Flexibility Exercise After proper warm up, hold gentle stretches for at least 30 seconds (no bouncing).

Balance Exercise Tai Chi, Yoga, or specific balance exercises can be very effective in reducing the risk of falling.

For health concerns ranging from muscle strength to brain function, from heart health to diabetes, regular exercise is the most important anti-aging advice these writings will have to offer.

Falls—the sixth leading cause of death in those ages 65 and older—are not just a function of muscle strength. Changes in the speed of nerve transmission affect both gross and skilled motor function. Fast twitch (speed) muscle fibers tend to atrophy at a higher rate than slow twitch (endurance) fibers, leading to slower reaction times and balance issues.

A drop in blood pressure to the head may also lead to a fall. When I get up from lying down (especially in the night when I am half asleep), I sit on the edge of the bed for a minute to make sure that my brain is ready to coordinate my journey to the bathroom. I give time for my blood pressure to adjust to the effects of gravity. Any dizziness or lightheadedhess may be a sign of insufficient blood flow for safety.

Let's be careful out there!

The Great Follicle Rebellion

My hair follicles are in revolt. Some have abandoned their post at the top of my head. Others are retreating from my hairline. Some of the deserters seem to have taken up crowded residence in my eyebrows where they pass the time growing long, crooked, gray hairs. Other follicles have sought shelter in my ears and nose. They have lost all discipline.

I remember as a teenager my hair was so thick the barber used thinning shears on it. Dark curls would litter the floor under my chair. I used to curse my hair. I could never comb the thick mass into the slick-back ducktail that was popular at the time. Only briefly in the '70s—when "white afros" were stylish—did I appreciate my hair. Now it is getting its revenge.

My father kept a full head of hair until the day he died. I expected to be granted the same fate, but the genetic shuffle had other plans. Instead, I inherited my mother's hair loss. She was nearly bald by her sixties. Fortunately for me, there has been some compromise. So far, my bald spot is limited to the top of my head. Good thing I am tall.

I did follow my father in another hair trait—turning gray early. It never bothered me. I always thought of it as "executive hair."

If you are over fifty and do not yet have gray hair, you are in the minority. Hair changes, particularly graying, are some of the first signs of aging. This may be an evolutionary strategy. Nature wants us to choose partners that give us the best chance of passing our DNA to future generations.

If we can tell age by appearance, it helps us select mating partners that are young and healthy—better able to protect and provide for offspring. When it comes to romance, our free will is tempered by nature's push to get our genes passed on. In response, we clever humans have invented hair color, hairpieces, wigs, and hair transplants to help us fool the instincts of our potential mates. Cosmetic interventions can be quite successful.

Just as men's self-image is tied to muscular strength, women's self-image is often tied to attractiveness. Changes in hair and skin may be particularly unsettling to "maturing" women. (Any further comment might be dangerous to my well-being.)

As a generation with a healthy number of tree-hugging, granola-munching nature enthusiasts, some of us are choosing to age without cosmetic intervention. "Natural" is consistent with our values.

As a generation that thinks of itself as eternally youthful, others among us are trying to hide any evidence to the contrary.

As the generation of "do your own thing," we embrace all choices.

****

Gray hair is the result of the progressive loss of *melanocytes* in hair bulbs (the base of growing hair). Melanocytes are cells that produce *melanin*, the pigment that gives color to our skin, eyes, and hair. There are two main types of melanin produced—one ranges from dark brown to black, the other red to yellow. Our hair color depends on the blend of these pigments as dictated by our genes.

As we age, fewer melanocytes are created. Thus, we produce less melanin and grayer hair. White hair has no melanin at all.

Hair grows out of skin structures called follicles. Scientists have found that hair follicles produce small amounts of hydrogen peroxide—a bleaching agent. In younger people, this is broken down by an enzyme called *catalase*. As we age, catalase production decreases, allowing hydrogen peroxide to interfere with melanin production. We essentially bleach the color out of our own hair.

We have all noticed how Presidents develop gray hair during their time in office. Can stress cause gray hair as folklore says? Researchers say yes—or at least maybe.

Evidence suggests that the sustained release of the neurotransmitters associated with the "fight or flight" response can cause DNA damage in melanocytes—reducing melanin production. With or without stress, we will all eventually produce gray hair. It is just a matter of timing.

Each of our 100,000+ strands of hair in the scalp normally grows for two to six years, enters a resting phase for several months, and then falls out. The average person looses about 100 scalp hairs a day. The cycle length for growth and replacement in a particular individual determines whether their hair can naturally grow to shoulder length or waist length. Eyelash and eyebrow hairs are short because they have a shorter growing cycle—they fall out before they get very long.

Although environmental factors (including radiation and nutritional deficiencies) can cause hair loss, over 80% is genetically controlled.
The most common type of hair loss is called *androgenetic alopecia*. This condition causes a disruption in the ordinary pattern of hair growth and replacement. Hair follicles construct shorter and thinner strands of hair—or stop hair growth altogether.

In men, this is "male-pattern baldness." It produces the characteristic receding hairline and thinning crown that can eventually join in complete baldness. Over half of the male population will experience some degree of male-pattern baldness by age fifty, 90% by age ninety.

In women, androgenetic alopecia produces general thinning but is much less common and rarely leads to complete baldness. This is because the male hormone testosterone stimulates the follicle changes that produce baldness.

The genetics of balding is quite complex, involving the variable expression of several genes. One of these genes is the *androgen receptor gene* (AR). This gene promotes the response of cells to testosterone and other hormones. Some variations of this gene contribute to androgenetic alopecia.

The AR gene is passed on the X chromosome. This means that males receive only one of these genes—from their mothers. Females receive two of these genes—one from each parent. Since females have two of the AR genes, they have an increased chance of having one that prevents baldness.

Before you men blame your mother for your hair loss, statistics show that those of you who have bald fathers are also at greater risk of baldness. Like I said, the genetics involved is complex. (Apologies to the high school biology teachers who tried to keep things simple.)

Some treatments for baldness are available, including Rogaine and Propecia. They are less than 50% effective in restoring some hair growth and do come with side effects.

We Boomers used to recognize each other by our long hair. Now we still recognized each other by our hair—gray or absent!

Elephant Skin

My skin is becoming more patriotic with age: bruises turn red, skin stays white, and varicose veins are blue.

I was stretching on the floor this morning with my leg straight in front of me when I did something I have never done before. I looked at the knee that lay just inches from my face. I mean, I really *looked* at it.

"This knee could belong to an elephant," I thought with some surprise. Hundreds of deep wrinkles form tight concentric circles around my kneecap. Crossing the plateau in the middle of this rugged terrain are more wrinkles, shallower and wider spaced. Some of these wrinkles form a pattern of diamond shapes. The pattern of all these crevices is interrupted by smooth islands of scar tissue—the results of dozens of cuts and scrapes suffered over the decades.

Closer examination revealed a landscape decorated with widely dispersed hairs, growing wild with every angular shape imaginable. Hairs on the kneecap are short and rare, becoming longer and denser in the surrounding circular fault zone. I must admit, I have never examined an elephant's knees closely, but it can't look much different.

Inspecting other areas of skin, I do notice one difference from elephants. My skin is thinner. In fact, it has become much thinner—and more vulnerable—as the years have passed. Not only does my paper skin tear easily, but it also bruises at the slightest provocation. Bump the back of my hand on the side of the washing machine as I remove clothes—I display a bruise for a week.

21

I extend my fingers and examine the back of my hand. It is a repulsive mass of rigid tendons with bulging blue-green veins crossing over and between them like some poorly planned irrigation system. Covering the unsightly mess is the thinnest of skin coatings folded into deep wrinkles between the tendons and veins. My God, my hands look like they belong to a centenarian.

When I was young, I was teased for my freckles. Now they have been replaced by every manner of colored splotches, ragged bumps, and rough patches. My dermatologist can name them all, but he has been kind enough to dismiss most of them by calling them "wisdom spots." More seriously, I have had six skin cancers already—including one life-threatening melanoma.

I know now that the sun is not my friend. We used to be close when I grew up in Southern California. Those were the days when tans were cool and sunscreens were for wimps. Our generation will suffer for our ignorance. Just compare the skin on your bottom with that from the sun-exposed parts of your body. The contrast is likely extreme. My butt skin looks and feels like it belongs to a baby (take my word).

I should have lived my life wrapped in aluminum foil.

Yes, the sunburns of youth have cost me. Now I see my dermatologist as regularly as I see my dentist. The peace of mind is worth it. My mother died of melanoma.

Skin is the façade that gives others their initial impression of us. Our first facial wrinkles are an unwelcome reminder that we are aging—and others can see it. The skin surrounding the eye is the thinnest in the body (.5 mm), thus often the first area to display wrinkles ("crow's feet").

22

In a culture that values the attractiveness of youth, reactions to skin changes can range from slight surprise to utter dismay. In any case, they are inevitable. Genetics and sun damage determine our fate.

The importance of protecting ourselves from the sun cannot be overemphasized. The Australians (who are at elevated risk because of a hole in the protective ozone layer above them) have a saying: "*Slip, Slop, Slap.*"

Slip on a shirt, **Slop** on the sunscreen, **Slap** on a hat.

Also, limit exposure between the hours of 10 and 4 when the sun's rays are most direct.

(Note: Damaging UVA rays *do* penetrate the side windows of cars! Skin damage—including cancer—is more likely on the left side of Americans who have driven a lot.)

Regular skin checks by a dermatologist or primary care physician can be potentially lifesaving. Self-checks (and partner checks) may help avoid nasty surprises.

****

The skin is the largest organ of the body, accounting for approximately 16% of total body weight. By age sixty-five, nearly half of all people will have some skin disorder that requires medical treatment.

Skin consists of three layers and aging has a negative effect on each of them.

The top layer of skin is the *epidermis*. These cells produce a fibrous substance called *keratin*. The outermost layer of the epidermis consists of dead cells filled with this protective, water resistant protein. In young skin, these dead cells are sloughed off and replaced every 15-30 days. This replacement rate is reduced by 50% by age seventy.

The reduction in the rate of skin cell replacement has several consequences. For one, wounds take longer to heal. This is a serious problem in the elderly. They become much more likely to suffer from skin infections, including bedsores during extended illnesses. The risk of skin cancer is also elevated because cells are exposed to the sun's radiation for longer periods before they are replaced.

As in hair follicles, melanocytes in epidermal cells produce our skin color. The number of melanocytes may be reduced by as much as 20% per decade after age thirty. This leads to irregular pigmentation ("age spots") and reduced tanning ability.

Other age-related changes in the epidermis include increased roughness and dryness. Older epidermis is less efficient at retaining moisture than young epidermis. This occurs at the same time that oil and sweat glands reduce their output. Dry skin may become cracked and irritated, leading to redness, itchiness, pain, and swelling. This condition is called *eczema* or *dermatitis*.

Over-the-counter moisturizers can help with dry skin and itching. Additionally, a dermatologist may prescribe skin medications and office treatments that may be very effective.

Below the epidermis is the *dermis*. This connective tissue is the "working" area of the skin, containing the hair follicles, sweat glands, oil glands, sense organs, and blood vessels. A protein called *collagen* provides significant structural support of this layer.

The total amount of collagen in the skin decreases about 1% a year after age twenty, producing a matching decrease in skin thickness. At the same time, structural changes in the collagen reduce its flexibility, making older skin more subject to tear-type injuries. (When I'm working with my hands, I often look down to find a bloody chunk of skin peeled back.)

Age-related changes in elastic fibers and collagen fibers in the dermis reduce the stretch and resilience of older skin. This produces the sagging and wrinkling that we associate with aging. Repeated extensions and compressions of the skin (as in smiling, laughing, squinting, etc.) cause damage to supportive fibers, which are not fully repaired. These damaged areas define our most noticeable wrinkles.

What can be done about wrinkles? Not as much as we might like. Despite advertising claims to the contrary, there is no scientific support for the effectiveness of over-the-counter moisturizers and skin creams to *prevent* wrinkles. They are helpful for combating dryness and may provide a modest and temporary improvement in appearance.

A dermatologist may offer a variety of options to reduce wrinkles, including Retin-A, glycosaminoglycans, dermal fillers, botulinum toxin, and laser resurfacing. Plastic surgery would be the extreme intervention.

Also in the dermis, receptors for both pressure and light touch decrease with age, potentially reducing fine motor performance with the hands. Nail growth slows with age, with nails becoming thinner and more brittle.

Under the dermis is the *subcutaneous fat layer*. It varies greatly in thickness as it performs its various functions of insulation, protection, and energy storage.

Thermoregulation is a common complaint among the elderly. A reduction in the number of blood vessels and sweat glands in the dermis makes cooling less efficient. Many older people are easily overheated.

At the other extreme, thinning skin, reduced fat, decreased muscle activity, and poor blood circulation can produce "chilling." (NO, you will never catch me in a cardigan sweater like my father used to wear around the house.)

Skin growths (my wife and I call them barnacles) are common among older people. Some examples include:

Age Spots   – flat, light brown, similar to large freckles.

Seborrheic Keratoses – dark, rough, irregular, "wart-like" bumps that may have a "stuck-on" look.

Actinic Keratoses – scaly or crusty, pink, red, tan, or brown spots.

Skin Tags   – soft, flesh-colored (or dark) bumps or skin extensions, often connected to the skin by a stalk.

<u>Cherry Angiomas</u> – overgrowths of blood vessels producing small raised red or purple bumps.

<u>Moles</u> – colored (usually dark), flat or raised, variety of shapes and sizes. *These occasionally give rise to the dangerous cancer melanoma.*

Moles should be professionally evaluated if they:
- are new or growing
- show changes, including roughness or bleeding
- have irregular or jagged edges
- contain several colors (tan, brown, black, red)

With many of us prone to denial, I introduce the following mantra:

If it doesn't look right, feel right, or work right—get it checked!

Call a Plumber

In the early summer of 2003, I began to notice chest pain when I went for my daily walks. It was more noticeable after I had eaten, so I decided I must be developing heartburn. I tried home remedies such as consuming smaller meals and taking antacids.

I still went on our long planned Alaskan cruise in July. The episodes of discomfort continued, but I was determined not to let it interfere with our vacation. I struggled through. Finally, it was time for departure from the ship. I felt a lot of stress—packing, moving luggage, worrying about plane flights, etc.

Suddenly I had the worst episode of "heartburn" I had experienced yet. I could barely breathe—it felt like an elephant was sitting on my chest. I was sweating and nauseated. The intense pain continued through our disembarkation, the bus ride to the airport, and the flight home. (Yes, it is appropriate at this point for you to say "What an idiot!" or some similar phrase.) Even with training in physiology and health education, I managed to maintain a state of complete denial.

Once home, I went to see my gastroenterologist. When I described my symptoms, I could see the color drain from his face. He handed me some nitroglycerine tablets and told me to take them if my symptoms returned. My problem, he said, was not digestive. It sounded like I had suffered a heart attack—and I should see a cardiologist *immediately*.

The cardiologist evaluated me on a treadmill. I lasted less than two minutes. He scheduled me for an angiogram.

The test revealed that my LAD (Left Anterior Descending) coronary artery was 100% blocked. This is the most important blood vessel feeding the heart muscle, sometimes called the "widow maker" because of the undesirable outcomes of blockages in this artery.

My doctor told me that the only reason I did not die (of my stupidity) was that I had developed collateral circulation to provide oxygen to the heart muscle. As the LAD had been slowly compromised by cholesterol deposits, extra coronary arteries had grown. My routine of daily walking had saved my life by encouraging supplemental blood vessel development.

The pain I felt at the end of the cruise was probably the rupture of a plaque (deposit) that had partially restricted the LAD for some time. This led to a blood clot that completely blocked the artery. (In my attempt at self-treatment for my "heartburn," I had stopped taking my daily aspirin that helps prevent blood clots. All of this is completely embarrassing for me. I share it in the hope that others may be saved.)

During angioplasty, my doctor had the skill to break through the blood clot in my LAD. With the blockage removed, he was able to install a stent to help keep it open. I was placed on medications to lower my blood pressure, prevent clots, and reduce my cholesterol. I am happy to report no more issues with "heartburn."

Coronary artery disease is the leading cause of death in America. I consider myself extremely lucky to be alive.

****

Even in healthy aging, the walls of arteries become thicker and less elastic. This can raise blood pressure. More than half of people age sixty-five or over have high blood pressure. Yet, most will be unaware of their condition unless tested because it rarely causes noticeable symptoms. Having blood pressure checked regularly is a simple, painless, and vital health practice.

The effects of high blood pressure are dangerous and cumulative. Persistent high blood pressure damages arteries, causing tiny fissures and rough surfaces on the interior that speed the buildup of deposits of cholesterol and other fatty materials. High blood pressure also can weaken arteries, enlarge the heart (a step toward heart failure), and damage the brain and kidneys.

If lifestyle changes (such as weight loss and reduced salt intake) do not bring blood pressure in line, many effective medications are available today. For example, *diuretics* increase the amounts of salt and water excreted by the kidneys, reducing blood volume. This means the heart does not have to work as hard and blood pressure is reduced. *Beta-blockers* slow the heart rate and lessen the force of the heart's contractions. *ACE inhibitors* dilate blood vessels, opening the pathway for blood to flow with less resistance. Some combination of these will usually be successful in lowering blood pressure to healthy levels.

Another life-threatening issue is the development of *arteriosclerosis*—hardening of the arteries. Some loss of artery elasticity is normal with aging, but lifestyle choices may accelerate the process. Arteriosclerosis can lead to the first and fourth leading cause of death in America: heart disease and stroke.

Atherosclerosis is a specific type of arteriosclerosis. It refers to the buildup of substances on the interior of artery walls. Atherosclerosis begins in childhood as cholesterol and fatty materials gradually stick to vessel walls to form deposits called *plaques*.

Over time, calcium accumulates in the plaques, causing blood vessels to become narrowed and stiff. The resulting reduced flow often remains asymptomatic until restriction reaches seventy percent.

These plaques can also burst, triggering a blood clot (*thrombi*) to form. This can block blood flow. If this happens in a coronary artery, oxygen is cut off from the heart muscle, resulting in a heart attack. If it happens in the brain, it may cause a stroke.

Aspirin has both an anti-inflammatory effect on artery walls and an anticoagulant effect on platelets (that help clot the blood). For these reasons, your doctor may recommend an aspirin regimen if risk factors for heart disease are present.

Despite all the negative press because of their relationship to heart disease, lipids (fats) play a vital role in the blood. Triglycerides are an important source of cell energy. Cholesterol is an essential part of cell membranes and is necessary for the production of many hormones. Other lipids help transport fat-soluble vitamins.

Nevertheless, an overabundance of some fats in the blood may have a significant impact on the development of atherosclerosis. The following lifestyle guidelines should be kept in mind:

** Eating excess calories contributes to high triglyceride levels (bad).
** Consuming saturated fats and trans fats raises LDL levels (bad).
** Regular exercise increases HDL levels (good).

Family history, age, and being male contribute to the risk of atherosclerosis. **Other risk factors can be controlled, including levels of cholesterol and other fats in the blood, high blood pressure, diabetes, tobacco smoking, excess weight, and physical inactivity.**

Although modern lifestyle may accelerate the condition, atherosclerosis has been found in ancient Egyptian mummies and described in early Greek writings. It is present in almost all animal species. Therefore, the issue is less about how to avoid atherosclerosis and more about how to manage it so it does not become life threatening.

Because our genetic makeup plays a major role, lifestyle changes alone may not bring blood fats into desirable ranges. In that case, medications like *statins* may be helpful. Statin drugs are very effective in regulating lipid levels in the blood if lifestyle modification is not successful.

Atherosclerosis does not have to be an inexorably progressive condition. This is one of the most hopeful clinical findings of the last twenty years. The key, in consultation with your doctor, is to do whatever is necessary to get your lipids in line. By making the right choices, including medications if necessary, our atherosclerosis can be stabilized—*or even reversed.*

Routine blood tests are thus a valuable tool in disease prevention. Your doctor will help you evaluate your test results, but the following guidelines will generally apply:

- Triglycerides should be below 150 mg/dL (after fasting).
- Low-density lipoprotein (LDL) cholesterol ideally should be less than 130 mg/dL. (Under 100 mg/dl is the goal for those with evidence of heart disease.) This is the "bad" cholesterol that forms the artery-clogging plaques.
- High-density lipoprotein (HDL) is best above 40 mg/dL (50 mg/dL in women). This cholesterol actually helps prevent atherosclerosis by removing LDL from the bloodstream.

Unfortunately, cardiovascular disease is still the number one killer of Americans. But let's again focus on the positive: death rates due to cardiovascular disease have decreased more than 50% in recent decades. Many of us have improved our lipid profile with diet and medications. We have lowered our blood pressure with weight management and medications. Our healthy aging choices to stop smoking, exercise more, and consume better foods have also been key.

In the 1990s it was shown that we can not only prevent athero-sclerosis, but *we can induce disease regression in arteries that are already affected.* This finding provides hope to all of us who seek healthy aging. The bottom line:

Lifestyle choices can reduce heart disease risk by 80%.

Researchers have noted that a particular combination of health risks dramatically increases the chances of coronary artery disease, stroke, and type 2 diabetes. They have labeled this collection of risk factors *Metabolic Syndrome*. Meeting most of the following goals allows an individual to reduce the risk of this health threatening condition:

-- Manage triglycerides, LDL, and HDL as listed above.

But also:

-- Avoid abdominal obesity (defined as 40-inch waistline for
    men and 35-inch for women).
-- Keep average blood pressure below 130 / 85 mm Hg.
-- Keep fasting blood glucose less than 100 mg/dL.

31

Even with perfect lifestyle choices and proper use of medications, the risk of heart attack will never be zero. Quick action—and overcoming denial—can save lives.

SYMPTOMS OF HEART ATTACK

- ➤ Uncomfortable pressure, squeezing, or pain in chest
- ➤ Pain in arm(s), jaw, back, neck, stomach
- ➤ Shortness of breath
- ➤ Cold sweat, lightheadedness, nausea/vomiting

Women are less likely to experience chest pain and more likely to experience shortness of breath, jaw pain, and nausea.

Nearly half of all heart attacks, for both men and women, are now thought to be silent—meaning they do not produce the classic chest pain and tightness. Therefore, if you experience *any* combination of these symptoms:

Don't wait—Call 911

That Egyptian River

Denial.

It is one of the most dangerous health challenges of aging. We don't want to admit that our body is changing—even though it is completely natural and should be expected. As evidenced in my last essay, my denial could have killed me.

Here is another story:

We were in the final days of an exploration of the Big Island of Hawaii in 2010. Circumnavigating in our rental car, we stopped for the night in several different regions. We hiked in the crater of a dormant volcano, watched the nightglow of a still-active Kilauea, and searched for new lava flows into the ocean. Our drive had taken us through scenery ranging from magnificent waterfalls in lush tropical rain forests on the wet side, to desolate moonscapes and deserted beaches on the dry side. Everything had gone perfectly.

We had planned to spend our last three days relaxing in a condominium near Kona. We wanted to soak up as much Aloha as possible before heading back to the mainland. Our condo had been carefully selected for its proximity to a beautiful spot called Magic Sands Beach.

We awoke to a picture postcard morning, the sun glistening off the turquoise blue water, the temperature comfortable, and the breezes gentle. After several days in the car, I was ready to enjoy the beach—and it was right next door.

We walked over with our towels and beach chairs. At this early hour, we practically had the idyllic scene to ourselves. A few locals were surfing the waves at the opposite end of the cove. Only two young families shared the white sand with us, and they were a good distance down the crescent shaped shore. Perfect.

I couldn't wait to get in the tropical water. The waves looked to be a gentle three feet or so. I told my wife that I was going to do some bodysurfing. As I walked to the water's edge, I felt young and invigorated. My mind was back in high school when I used to love bodysurfing the waves in Huntington Beach. When I entered the water, it was pleasantly warmer than it had ever been in Southern California. Perfect.

After a couple of aborted attempts, I caught a small wave and rode it for a dozen yards before it petered out. I was conscious that my wife, Carolyn, might be watching me from shore, so I turned quickly to go back out and catch a better wave.

Soon a bigger set was approaching. I rode up and over the first wave and got into position to catch the second. I didn't want to fail on this attempt, so I swam with everything I had. Just at the last second, as the wave started to break, I could feel myself being sucked into it. I was elated that I had caught the wave—for a fraction of a second.

When I looked down, I could tell that the first wave had already retreated, taking most of the water out with it. I realized I was going "over the falls" into shallow water—the surfer's nightmare—and there was nothing I could do to stop myself.

I had gone over the falls many times as a young man. Back then, I could curl into a ball and ride it out. Sometimes it felt like being in a washing machine, but I always came out unscathed.

This time, when the wave pushed me down, I didn't have the flexibility or strength to curl quickly. There was an audible, sickening crack as my head slammed into the sand. The jolt stunned me. The pain told me it was bad.

When I tried to stand, I realized I could not hold up my head. I had to grab it on both sides with my hands as I struggled to walk out of the water. I was scared.

When I reached Carolyn, I said: "We need to go to the emergency room." We walked back to the condo, with me holding my head up by hand.

I would like to blame shock for my next decision, but if I am honest, it is another entry in the denial column. I should have called 911 right from the beach. Failing that, I should have called 911 from our condo. Instead, I told my wife that I needed to take a shower before going to the hospital. My scalp was bleeding, and wet sand covered me from head to toe. So holding my head up with my hands, I tried to rinse off some of the sand. This decision could have paralyzed me if I had damaged a spinal nerve.

We got in the car. Carolyn said she had found the hospital on her phone's GPS mapping app. We followed the instructions, only to discover that the road suggested did not go through. We had to turn around and start over. Calling 911 definitely would have been a better option.

When we finally arrived at the emergency room, the receptionist immediately put me in a neck brace. It felt so good to have my head supported.

She asked me what happened and I explained about my mishap on Magic Sands Beach. She said, "We call it Tragic Slams Beach. We get someone like you here every week."

My snarky self thought: *That unmarked beach must be good for emergency room business.* But truthfully, I should have examined the wave action more carefully before "taking the plunge."

X-rays showed that I had fractured my C-5 neck vertebrae. The doctor was concerned that swelling might cause nerve damage, and they did not have a neurosurgeon to respond to such an issue on The Big Island. I would have to be life-flighted to Honolulu.

You would think $25,000 would have gotten me a more comfortable ride. I was too tall for the gurney and they barely managed to squeeze me into the small ambulance plane.

A couple of days later, when they decided I was stable, Carolyn and I flew back to the mainland. After several months in a neck brace and a couple more of rehab, I was told: "Go forth and do not sin (bodysurf) again."

Perhaps the biggest insult to my ego came when I received my case notes from the hospital in Honolulu. They started with the words:

"An elderly gentleman presented with..."

The Domino Effect

One early morning in 2012, I plopped myself on the couch to do some reading. The house was quiet as I sat sideways with my legs outstretched, adjusting a pillow behind my back. Shortly after I began to read, I simultaneously heard and felt something in my chest—like the sloshing of a washing machine. In the next instant, I could not breathe.

I rolled onto all fours on the floor and gasped for air. I felt as if I was suffocating and complete panic set it. It was the worst feeling I have ever had. I thought I might be dying.

I managed to call out my wife's name. When she entered the room, I told her "Can't breathe—call 911." I continued to gasp for air and thought I might pass out. Part of me wanted to pass out, but I was afraid I would never wake up.

The next few minutes seemed eternal, but the sound of a distant siren was comforting. Paramedics immediately put me on oxygen, which helped. Maybe I won't die, I thought.

On the way to the hospital, I heard the paramedic call ahead. My pulse, blood pressure, and ECG (EKG) were normal. I wondered if he thought I was faking it.

The initial emergency room exam confirmed that I was not having a heart attack. After a chest X-ray, the doctor gave me the diagnosis: *bilateral pulmonary embolism.*

"You are very fortunate," the doctor said. "Up to thirty percent of people who have a pulmonary embolism do not survive." He explained that a blood clot had come loose somewhere in my body and had broken up as it passed through my heart. The pieces had then simultaneously blocked several of the pulmonary arteries in my lungs.

37

He immediately started me on blood thinners and sent me to an ultrasound technician to search for the source of the original blood clot. When all the testing was completed, the story came together. I had been the victim of *the domino effect*.

As I described in the previous essay, two years earlier I managed to break my neck while bodysurfing in Hawaii. After a year of recovery, my body was not in great shape. I had been sitting around for several months, much of it with a neck brace on. I was just beginning to walk regularly.

Meanwhile, several people in our community had begun to play pickleball, a tennis-like game using a smaller court. Once again, I made an ill-advised choice. (You may detect a pattern here.) Just as I thought I could body surf Hawaii with the strength and flexibility I had as a teenager, I thought I could walk on the pickleball court and instantly return to my athletic glory days. Within the first few minutes of playing, I lunged for a ball and heard an audible pop. Down I went. Having suffered my share of athletic injuries when I was young, I knew this was serious.

There was less pain than I expected, but I discovered I could not flex my left foot. It was obvious to me that I had torn my Achilles' tendon. An urgent care physician easily confirmed the diagnosis. It was a complete rupture. There was no longer any connection between my calf muscle and the back of my heel.

Within a week, I was on the operating table having my tendon surgically repaired. This meant more months of recovery.

Fast forward, and a year later I am on the floor of my living room, gasping for air.

A blood clot that had formed during my Achilles surgery or recovery had broken free in a leg vein and nearly killed me. See the domino effect? Broken neck → torn Achilles → deep vein thrombosis → pulmonary embolism.

It is common for a fall, illness, or other health event to trigger more issues down the road. The key is to allow time for a full recovery, completing any rehab prescribed. Remain as active as your condition allows. Then restart your normal activities slowly—mindful that it can take a while to return to your previous levels of health and fitness. This can be a time of vulnerability.

In my case, I wish I had been more aware of the dangerous potential of blood clots. Only later did I learn that differences in structure make blood clots more likely in the left leg than the right. I also wish I had insisted on blood thinning medications and compression stockings following my surgery.

If I had understood the risks, perhaps I could have avoided my life and death experience with pulmonary embolism. I am glad I did not die so I could live and learn.

****

The formation of a blood clot in a vein is called *deep vein thrombosis* (DVT). They most often occur in the muscles and tissues of the calves and thighs. Unlike arteries that are constructed with their own muscle layer to push the blood along, veins rely on the contraction of surrounding body muscles to propel blood back to the heart. This means that inactivity allows the blood to pool, sometimes resulting in blood clots.

When a person is not contracting their leg muscles, like on a long flight or when bedridden, DVT is a particular threat. It can also occur following surgery or leg injury.

Deep vein thrombosis often occurs with few or no symptoms. If there are symptoms, they may include deep aching pain or swelling in the leg.

As we become seniors, it is even more important to be aware of stretching and standing at least every two hours when traveling. Adequate hydration is essential. Elastic stockings may be advisable.

Pneumatic stockings (that contract) and blood thinners may be appropriate for those requiring extended bed rest. If your doctor does not discuss it with you, bring up your concerns with your doctor.

The prevention of blood clots (DVTs) is crucial to guard against life-threatening pulmonary embolism.

Breathing Is a Good Thing

Bad news: lung function naturally decreases with age. Total surface area of air sacs declines, respiratory muscles weaken, and elasticity of lung structures decreases.

Good news: the total loss of function is normally not enough to interfere with daily tasks. The average person in their seventies maintains over 75% of the lung capacity they had in their youth. However, vigorous exercise or high altitude can betray the changes.

Other major lung problems besides pulmonary embolism include cancer, pneumonia, and *COPD*. *Chronic Obstructive Pulmonary Disease* is a general term for reduced capacities in air passages of the lungs. Over 16 million Americans have some form of COPD. Reduced smoking rates and decreased exposure to air pollution should help more of us Boomers escape COPD.

Emphysema is one example of COPD. It is a debilitating and scary condition that most often results from smoking. It occurs when the walls of tiny air sacs (*alveoli*) that comprise the lungs degenerate. As healthy lung tissue disappears, airflow and gas exchange are reduced in proportion. There is just less lung tissue to do the job.

Chronic Bronchitis is the other major form of COPD. In this case, airflow is reduced as the walls of airways (*bronchioles*) swell, spasm, and fill with mucus.

COPD increases the chances of dangerous lung infections like pneumonia. Lung infections are among the top ten leading causes of death in the United States.

As we age, lung infections become ever more life threatening because our immune function declines, our cough reflex weakens, and the natural lung cleaning movement of cilia and mucus slows. After age fifty, the incidence of respiratory disease steadily increases. Yet, even after age eighty-five, an individual has a 75% chance of *not* dying of lung disease.

Every chance I get, I take a deep breath—gratefully!

****

Pneumonia is an infection of the small air sacs of the lungs and surrounding tissue. Bacteria are the most common infectious agents, but viruses and fungi cause some cases. The pathogens that cause pneumonia are everywhere and we inhale them all the time. The decline in immune competence with age explains why pneumonia is a serious, life-threatening problem for the elderly.

Antibiotics are usually effective against bacteria. Antiviral drugs combat viruses. (They are most effective if given in the first day or two after symptoms appear.)

Fortunately, today we have a pneumonia vaccine. Older people should check with their health care provider to make sure that their vaccinations are up to date.

Influenza (flu) is another disease that is dangerous in the elderly, causing over 15,000 deaths of older Americans each year. Pneumonia is the primary cause of death resulting from influenza infection. While not perfect, the flu vaccine can substantially reduce the chances of both contracting and dying from the flu. Because the flu virus mutates from year to year, the updated flu vaccine must be taken annually.

If an older person has trouble breathing, immediate medical treatment is imperative. (High fever and confusion are often associated symptoms of pneumonia.)

Us Against the World

We are constantly under attack. Parasites would like to invade us. Bacteria would like to use us as a food source. Viruses would like to enter our cells to reproduce. The battle is ongoing. Only when an invader temporarily gets the upper hand do we say we are "sick."

Even when we are "healthy," we play host to trillions of bacteria, more than 1% of our body weight. That is enough to fill a half-gallon jug. Ugh! In fact, there are likely ten times as many bacteria cells in us as there are our own cells. (Bacteria cells are much smaller than body cells.) We host over 1,000 different bacterial species. We are walking Petri dishes!

Most of this microbiota is found in our intestines, but the surfaces of our body (including skin, mouth, throat, nose, etc.) are also covered with bacteria. Fortunately, most bacteria are harmless. Many actually provide valuable benefits including the production of vitamins and keeping harmful bacteria and fungi in check.

Our immune system evolved to protect us from attack from within and without. The central component of the immune system is a variety of white blood cells. Some are able to recognize foreign invaders and engulf them. Others produce chemicals called *antibodies* that can attach to the surface of germs and disable them.

A subset of white blood cells has the ability to remember invaders so that a quick response can be mounted to a subsequent invasion attempt. This is called *immunity*.

We acquire natural immunity when we fight off a disease, as many of us did with mumps, measles, and chicken pox. We usually have these diseases only once.

We can also develop artificial immunity by vaccination. Vaccines introduce dead or disabled *pathogens* (disease-causing organisms) into our bodies to allow our immune system to "practice" fighting against them. Our white blood cells then remember the shape of the pathogen's surface, allowing a quick response should the real thing invade our body at a future time.

Vaccination is not just for kids. Seniors can protect themselves by keeping their shots up to date (tetanus, pneumonia, flu, shingles, etc.)

In the rare cases when our immune system fails us, physicians have an arsenal of antibiotics that kill bacteria. These should *only* be used when needed and according to directions. (Finish prescriptions to prevent the development of resistant strains of bacteria.)

Our disease-fighting immune system is an elaborate and elegant mechanism that usually serves us well. As with other systems of the body, however, it becomes less efficient and reliable as we age. Sometimes it can even turn against us and produce *autoimmune* disorders such as arthritis and lupus. In these cases, our immune system becomes confused, attacking our own body cells as if they were foreign invaders.

****

In one theory of aging (*antagonistic pleiotropy theory*), natural selection has favored genes that confer short-term survival at the cost of increased deterioration later in life. Our immune system provides an excellent example.

In our youth, white blood cells produce antibodies and inflammatory responses to protect us from invasion by pathogens. This keeps our body healthy and strong, allowing us to reproduce and pass on our DNA.

As we age, the white blood cells that produce antibodies to foreign invaders decrease. This makes us more susceptible to serious infections like pneumonia and influenza. (Nature is not as worried about us after we have passed on our DNA.)

At the same time, the number of white blood cells that mistakenly react to our own body cells increases. This makes us more prone to autoimmune disorders such rheumatoid arthritis, systemic lupus. multiple sclerosis, and celiac disease.

As the name implies, autoimmune disorders occur when our usually efficient white blood cells make the serious error of reacting to our own body cells as if they were foreign invaders. This damages tissues, causes inflammation, and interferes with healthy function.

Inflammation is the swelling, redness, and warmth that we notice around a wound. In an attempt to protect the body, blood vessels expand to allow rapid transport to the area. Chemical messengers are released that attract an army of white blood cells. In addition, fluid is retained to help isolate the problem from the rest of the body. Inflammation also occurs internally where we may not be aware of it.

An acute episode of inflammation terminates when the cause of the problem is resolved. When the cause is ongoing, the inflammation becomes chronic and begins to damage surrounding tissues. Examples include over-exercising that stresses muscles, tendons and joints; overeating that stress the digestive and glandular systems; and autoimmune reactions.

Chronic inflammation is a strong contributor to atherosclerosis and the related risks of heart attack and stroke. It is also implicated in many other health concerns, including digestive issues, immune compromise, and some forms of cancer. A protective immune system that helps us survive in youth may turn against us in old age.

The damaging effects of chronic inflammation are well documented. What is less clear is how to control it. Removing an identified stressor is the first step—changing patterns of exercise or eating for example. Moderate, consistent exercise such as walking or swimming may actually have an anti-inflammatory effect. Conversely, overexertion ("weekend warrior") may add to damaging inflammation.

Anti-inflammatory drugs (NSAIDs) may seem like a logical answer, but the possibility of serious side effects reduce the attractiveness of this option. A risk–reward calculation in consultation with your doctor is wise.

Antioxidant supplementation (vitamins C, E or A for example) has been touted as anti-inflammatory. This sounds good in theory, but no clear clinical benefit has been shown. Some worrisome side effects *are* known. Eating vitamin-rich fruits and vegetables, however, is always safe and healthy.

The use of supplemental vitamins and herbs is an area ripe with misleading advice. They are advertised as fixes for every aspect of aging, ranging from heart disease and cancer prevention to the cure for colds and flu. Most are ineffective, and some are dangerous. (Thanks to intense lobbying by the industry, *the FDA cannot regulate supplements for their safety or effectiveness!*) Look to respected non-commercial sources of information and discuss supplementation with your doctor.

Note: The Baby Boom demographic has always made us a target for intense marketing. If you can sell to Boomers, you can get rich!

As we move into our senior years, purveyors of nutritional supplements, diets, exercise regimens, drugs, and cosmetic surgery are salivating. We need to do our homework. If we succumb to our desire for easy health fixes, we likely waste our time and money— possibly damaging our health as well. Let's be smart!

Stiffness Is Rarely a Good Thing

In addition to being called "elderly" at sixty-two (when I still thought of myself as middle-aged), the medical feedback generated during my "domino" events depressed me in another way. Every X-ray report I received at that time included a comment about the presence of *arthritis*. I had never really considered it. I had the common stiffness and pains of aging, but I had never specifically been diagnosed with arthritis. I should not have been so surprised.

arthro = joint, *itis* = inflammation

A minority of us will remain completely unaffected by arthritis. Even by age eighty, a fortunate 15% will completely escape it. Of course, that means the vast majority will have to deal with its effects, which range from annoying aches to severe disability. The label "arthritis" describes several different conditions, including osteoarthritis and rheumatoid arthritis.

Osteoarthritis is a chronic disorder of the cartilage, bones, and other joint tissues. It is sometimes called degenerative arthritis because the primary cause is wear and tear on the joints. Although there is a strong hereditary component, chronic overuse, injury, obesity, and high impact athletics all may contribute to its development.

Rheumatoid arthritis only affects 1% of the population. It often begins before age fifty. The cause of RA is unclear, but it is likely a form of autoimmune disease influenced by family genetics. In RA, the body's immune system attacks connective tissue lining the joints, eventually causing long-term damage. The disease is marked by flare-ups followed by periods of remission. Flare-ups are often accompanied by fatigue and low-grade fever.

Also found in joints are tendons (connecting muscle to bone) and bursae (fluid-filled sacs that cushion joint movement). Inflammation of these structures is labeled *tendonitis* or *bursitis*, respectively.

Distressingly, I am noticing the increasing effects of arthritis. My gait is not as smooth as it was, and it is difficult to stand erect when I first get out of a chair. These facts increase my motivation to keep stretching—and stay active.

****

Cartilage normally provides a cushion between bones at the joints. Osteoarthritis is an inflammation that occurs when cartilage becomes pitted and rough, promoting the development of tiny cavities in the bones beneath the cartilage. In severe cases, the end of the bone becomes irregular or bony outgrowths develop.

When we have osteoarthritis, temporary lack of movement commonly causes the joint to become stiff and painful. This may gradually ease when the joint is used (warmed up), but overuse or stressing the joint may increase pain. As the disease progresses, fluid may accumulate in the joints causing swelling. Some joints may eventually become enlarged and deformed.

A careful management plan may slow damage and reduce pain. Losing as little as eleven pounds can reduce the risk of osteoarthritis in the knees by 50%. Activities that put stress on joints should be limited. Exercises that strengthen surrounding muscles and ligaments may help improve joint function and reduce irritation.

As mentioned in the previous essay, nonsteroidal anti-inflammatory drugs (NSAIDs) reduce inflammation and relieve pain. Don't be fooled just because they are "over the counter" drugs. Their use should be discussed with your physician because they have important side effects in some people, including bleeding and increased risk of heart attack.

The Glasses Menagerie

I have become a collector of eyeglasses. I don't collect them for their style. I don't collect them because I lack awareness of where I can donate them. I collect them because I need them. Here is the story.

I first discovered I needed glasses back in high school. Reflecting on it now, I probably needed them much earlier. I guess I thought everyone was looking at the same fuzzy world that I was. Somehow, my vision—or lack thereof—only became an issue when I approached my sixteenth birthday and wanted to get my driver's license.

I remember vividly the drive home from the optometrist's office wearing my first pair of glasses. Everything was so clear and three-dimensional. Everything popped. I could read street signs and billboards from a block away. I could see the items for sale in store windows. It was a revelation.

At school, I could recognize faces from a distance and say hi to people that I had previously passed unrecognized.(They must have thought I was so stuck up or unfriendly.) Good vision was a game changer for this shy guy with limited social skills.

I even wore my new glasses to basketball practice. Up to this point, I had been shooting the ball at an ill-defined orange blob of a rim. Now I could actually see a basket with three dimensions. Soon I was wearing contact lenses for sports. I have been wearing glasses or contacts all of my adult life.

I have *myopia*—standard nearsightedness—a genetic gift from my father. In my mid-forties, I began to have trouble reading with my contacts in. I switched to monovision— wearing a contact for distance in one eye and one for reading in the other. It worked perfectly. I could see the faces of the kids in the back of my classroom and still read from the textbook on my desk. My brain adapted to the seeming confusion in a matter of days.

At the same time, I purchased a pair of bifocals to use when I was not wearing my contacts. I almost killed myself the first time I tried to walk down stairs. Once again, my brain soon adapted.

Everything went along perfectly until my sixties. Then I faced new challenges. I noticed that when I sat at the computer screen, neither the distance nor reading portion of my glasses produced an easy to read text. My ophthalmologist informed me that the ability of my lens to accommodate was just declining. She suggested that I get a pair of glasses set just for the distance between my computer monitor and my eyes. So it began.

My menagerie of glasses, in color-coded cases, now includes: everyday bifocals, computer glasses, mid-range bifocals (for playing cards), indoor sports glasses (not bifocals), outdoor dark sports glasses (not bifocals), dark bifocals (for driving).

Don't email me about progressive (multifocal) lenses. I added my first pair to the menagerie yesterday.

****

Eye changes are one of the first signs of aging. Usually, between the ages of forty and fifty, the lens in the eye stiffens. It becomes difficult to focus on objects that are closer than about two feet away. The standard joke is, "I can see fine, it is just that my arms are too short."

The reduction in the eye's ability to focus is called *presbyopia*. Reading glasses solve the problem. Those who already wear glasses for distance vision will get bifocals or multifocal lenses.

Other changes also occur to the lens of an aging eye. In addition to losing its flexibility, it tends to become denser. This lets less light through to the retina at the back of the eye. On average, sixty-year-olds need three times as much light to read as twenty-year-olds. (Try reading menus by candlelight!)

Older eyes have trouble adapting to rapid changes from light to dark or dark to light. This is because the muscles that widen and narrow the pupil are weaker and react more slowly. This can be especially important for night driving or for negotiating tunnels.

One disconcerting experience of aging is the increase in tiny black specks that move across the field of vision. These "floaters" are bits of solidified fluid and other debris inside the eye. They usually do not interfere with normal vision and are only a concern if they increase dramatically in a short period. In that case, an immediate professional examination is vital to check for vision-threatening problems with the retina.

A *cataract* is the clouding of the lens of the eye caused by changes in its structural proteins. It produces progressive, painless vision loss. The likelihood of developing cataracts increases steadily with age. Exposure to sunlight is thought to be a contributing factor, so the consistent use of sunglasses may help prevent or delay cataract development.

Fortunately, when cataracts affect safety, comfort, or the ability to perform daily tasks, they can usually be removed with surgery. In cataract surgery, the doctor makes a small incision in the eye, breaks up the cataract in the lens with ultrasound, and then removes the pieces. The capsule that surrounds the lens is left in place so that an artificial lens can be inserted to substitute for the natural lens. Complications are infrequent.

Glaucoma is a potential cause of blindness. It is a buildup of fluid pressure inside the eye that can damage the optic nerve. Since it is usually painless and produces no symptoms, older people should have comprehensive eye examinations every year or two.

Age-Related Macular Degeneration is a deterioration in the central and most sensitive part of the retina. It distorts vision and gradually results in a blind spot in one or both eyes. Although some peripheral vision may remain, activities such as reading and driving may become impossible.

The exact cause of Macular Degeneration is unknown, but family history, poor nutrition, and smoking are thought to increase the probability. A comprehensive eye exam may detect the early stages before symptoms become apparent. Treatments vary depending on the form of the disease and its stage of progression.

Many other conditions such as diabetic retinopathy, blood flow problems, and detached retina may threaten vision. My father experienced the sudden loss of vision in one eye (accompanied by "fireworks" and "floaters"), but did not seek immediate medical help. As a result, it was impossible to repair the detached retina that might otherwise have been surgically corrected. He lost the vision in that eye.

In summary: Anytime you experience rapid changes in your vision (partial or complete vision loss, "fireworks," excessive floaters, pain, etc.) seek immediate medical evaluation. Even if your vision seems fine, get a routine eye exam annually (a dilated eye exam—not just a glasses check).

Eyes are too important to risk.

(You may have noticed that I have used a slightly larger font than is normally found in paperback books. You're Welcome!)

What Did You Say?

Unlike my vision, so far my hearing has remained good. (My wife might occasionally disagree.) I will admit that it is sometimes difficult for me to follow conversations in a noisy environment, which is a definite sign of beginning hearing loss.

Some structures in the ear involved in hearing and balance naturally deteriorate with age. Atherosclerosis (caused by high cholesterol) can be a contributing factor.

By far, the most common cause of hearing loss is loud noise (shop equipment, jet engines, rock music, etc.). Repeated exposure gradually destroys the small hair-like projections that conduct sound in the cochlea of the ear. This damage is usually imperceptible at the time and accumulates for decades before hearing loss becomes apparent.

The auditory receptor cells in the ear's cochlea are established at birth—with no regeneration later in life. Thus, any damage to these cells is permanent.

We live in a 55+ community. A good percentage of our neighbors have developed hearing loss. Some have accepted it and use hearing aids. Others have not yet admitted any problem. It is easy to tell the difference.

Less than 40% of Americans with significant hearing loss use hearing aids, even though they can improve the quality of life for 95% of those that use them. (More denial?)

Cochlear implants are also an option in some cases.

****

By age sixty-five, 71% of the population have no significant hearing loss. This drops to 50% by age eighty. High-pitched sounds are usually the first ones that cause difficulty. The voices of women and children may thus be more difficult to hear than the base tones of a male.

Those with beginning hearing loss may accuse others of mumbling. This is because the consonants such as C, K, P, S, and T are quick, high-pitched sounds. Vowels are longer, lower pitched sounds. The inability to hear the consonant sounds in a sentence makes the words sound mumbled. Speaking louder does not help much because the vowels become louder, but not the consonants.

Earwax is also more likely to accumulate in older people, interfering with sound transmission. Normally, this oily substance is produced by glands in the ear canal to help protect against infections, much like mucus in the nose. With aging, both the earwax and the epidermis of the canal become dryer, causing earwax to stick to the walls. Non-prescription wax softening preparations are available to help dissolve and flush excess wax. (Never use objects to scrape inside the ear. Even cotton-tipped swabs may perforate the eardrum or cause infections.)

Tinnitus is often described as "ringing in the ear," although the sound may take many forms from hissing to buzzing to roaring. There are many causes, including hearing loss, fluid in the ear, atherosclerosis, and high doses of aspirin. In many cases, the cause is unknown. Fortunately, about 75% of people over age sixty-five do not report this condition.

Silencing the sounds of tinnitus is frequently difficult, but attempting to determine the cause is the first step. If correcting the cause is not possible, techniques can be employed to make the condition more bearable.

In all cases of hearing loss, a visit with an ear, nose, and throat specialist (ENT or otolaryngologist) is recommended for a complete workup of treatment options.

Syncopated Beat

When I was eleven or twelve years old, my Boy Scout troop was preparing for an extended backpacking trip on the John Muir Trail in the Sierra Nevada Mountains. My mother took me to the doctor to have a required physical.

Perhaps because of some bad experiences at age six when I had my tonsils removed, I was afraid of doctors. When our family physician placed his stethoscope on my chest, my heart was racing. The longer he listened, the faster my heart beat. After spending an extended time listening in several places on my chest and back, the doctor turned and asked my mom if she would kindly step outside of the room with him.

I am sure the doctor's discretion in not talking in front of me was designed to protect me. It had the opposite effect. My imagination went wild. I assumed I was dying.

On the way home, my mother explained that the doctor had heard a "heart murmur—a possible leaky valve." She told me that my heart had been beating so fast that the doctor could not be sure, so we were going to have some more tests done at the hospital. In my mind I heard, "You are dying."

The public hospital in downtown Los Angeles was a large institution that reeked of odd odors. It was crowded with unfamiliar people of every age, race, and ethnicity. I also knew the doctor had sent me there because I was dying. The whole situation was intensely frightening to me.

As we found our way to each testing department, mom would stand in line to check in, and then we would sit in a crowded room and wait. It took us half a day to get a chest X-Ray. (I had to swallow some disgusting thick liquid.) It seemed like another half a day to get an ECG. I do not remember how many tests we took or doctors we saw, but I know we spent at least two or three uncomfortable days there.

When we finally returned to our family physician, he said that the tests showed I had a slight heart murmur. He tried to reassure me that it was not unusual for a boy growing as fast as I was. He also said that I would probably outgrow it. What I heard was "Yes, you are dying."

By the time the doctor was prepared to sign my physical, it was too late for me to go on the hike. Instead, that summer I stayed at home and listened to my heart. I grew acutely aware of my heartbeat, especially when I lay in bed before going to sleep.

The awareness of my heartbeat has stayed with me throughout my life. For example, I hear and feel every time my heart skips a beat—commonly called a heart palpitation. My current cardiologist was amazed that I had heard and felt the blood clot sloshing through my heart before I had my pulmonary embolism.

Over the years, when I have been under extended stress, my palpitations have become chronic and bothersome. Even though my doctors have affirmed that they are normal and nothing to worry about, I sometimes still wonder if I am dying. Fortunately, since I retired from teaching, they have all but disappeared.

One night a couple of years ago, I awoke with a shortness of breath and a racing heart. I could feel that something was not normal. When it continued into the morning, I told my wife we had better go to the ER.

It did not take long for them to determine that I was having *atrial fibrillation*—rapid contractions of the upper heart chambers. Of course, I thought I was dying. Eventually, someone mentioned that atrial fibrillation is not usually life threatening. That was reassuring, but I was still stressed.

I was admitted to the hospital. They started an IV to give me medications to slow my heart rate and prevent blood clots. My cardiologist said he would come to the hospital to "convert" me. The nurse said this might involve either medications or giving my heart an electric shock to bring it back into normal rhythm.

After a couple of hours, the nurse said my cardiologist had notified her that he was on his way. I told her I had better go to the restroom before he arrived.

When I returned a few minutes later, I happily told the nurse that my normal heart rhythm had returned. She confirmed my observation and was amazed. She told me I was her first patient to have a spontaneous "bagal cardioversion." I later learned that she actually said "vagul cardioversion." My straining in the bathroom had stimulated the vagus nerve (the relaxation nerve), and that had brought my heart rhythm back to normal.

I have since learned that there are several ways to stimulate the vagus nerve. I have had three more episodes of afib and have been able to resolve each at home.

****

Normal heart rhythm is 60 to 80 beats per minute. Well-conditioned athletes may have a slower pulse (because their heart pumps more efficiently). Of course, heart rate increases with physical activity or stress. Unusually fast, slow, or irregular heart rhythms become more likely with age.

Palpitations—skipped beats, hard beats, irregular beats—are common and usually of no concern. Some people (like this frightened Boy Scout) find them worrisome while others barely notice them. They may have a variety of causes including exercise, excitement, anxiety, or chemical stimulants (caffeine, pseudoephedrine). Only rarely are they symptomatic of heart disease. If they are bothersome or cause symptoms such as chest pain or dizziness, they should be professionally evaluated.

Other types of arrhythmia are more likely to be of serious concern. *Atrial fibrillation* is the most common type of arrhythmia. It occurs when the top chambers of the heart (*atria*) lose their normal rhythm, contracting irregularly or rapidly. The condition may occur briefly or occasionally, only becoming chronic in about 10% of people over 80.

Because blood does not flow normally through the heart during atrial fibrillation, it increases the chance of blood clot formation. These blood clots may travel to the brain and cause a stroke. People with a tendency for atrial fibrillation are usually placed on blood-thinning medications such as warfarin (Coumadin) to reduce the risk of stroke.

Because the lower chambers of the heart (*ventricles*) pump blood to the entire body and lungs, disturbances in their contraction rhythms can be life threatening. In *ventricular tachycardia,* the heartbeats are regular but too rapid for proper blood flow. This can lead to dizziness, loss of consciousness, and heart failure. Sometimes heart rate can reach two hundred beats per minute. Even if it does not produce serious symptoms, this is still an extremely dangerous situation that requires immediate medical attention.

Old Horses

In many areas, life has come full circle. When I was three years old, my urination was a tinkle. I could create delicate golden patterns that sparkled on top of the toilet water. As a mature man, the goal was to sound as much like a horse as possible. A thunderous waterfall was a macho expression of manliness.

Now I am tinkling again.

Despite the emotional insult to my manhood, intellectually, I understand. Maximum urine volume in the bladder decreases with age, as does strength of bladder muscles. Then there is the pesky prostate that enlarges in all mature men and tends to partly block the flow of urine—a definite design failure on nature's part.

My internist always checks for PSA levels in my annual blood test. *Prostate Specific Antigen* is part of the seminal fluid produced by the prostate gland. A small amount of PSA makes its way into the blood. The amount varies linearly with the size of the prostate. Thus, PSA levels are used as an indicator of enlarged prostate and prostate cancer.

A few years ago, my PSA levels increased slightly above the 4 ng/mL level that is considered normal. My doctor sent me to a urologist. I had read a great deal about false positive PSA tests and the potential side effects of prostate biopsies and treatments. I was looking forward to a thorough discussion of my situation with an expert.

It was several weeks before I could get in to see the urologist. When the day of my appointment finally arrived,

I noticed a $200,000 luxury car in the parking spot labeled "Doctor Only." The office was large, well furnished, and professionally decorated. I was surprised by the number of staff bustling behind the counter. I thought, *this doctor is doing well.*

Before the urologist had even entered the exam room, his assistant came in and asked me when I wanted to schedule my biopsy. *What?* I couldn't believe it. No discussion of my particular situation. No discussion of side effects such as nerve damage or sexual dysfunction. *No discussion at all!* I told the assistant that I would not be scheduling a biopsy today. He seemed disappointed—like a car salesman when you say you are just looking.

I wondered if the words "up selling" were used in staff meetings. I could imagine a graph showing the number of procedures scheduled by each assistant during the month. Was a trip to Hawaii on the line?

When the doctor finally entered the room, I told him I knew that PSA tests were notorious for false positives, and I wanted to take a very conservative approach. He said I could safely wait a couple of months and have the test again. Two months later, my PSA levels were right back to normal.

I couldn't help but think of all the men who had undergone an unnecessary biopsy in this office. Being informed helped me dodge a bullet (or at least a long needle).

****

Benign Prostatic Hyperplasia (BPH) is the medical term for enlargement of the prostate gland. The prostate starts out the size of a walnut and is located just under the bladder where it surrounds the *urethra* (urine tube). It is tasked with producing fluids that become part of the semen.

Unlike any other internal organ, the prostate continues to grow until death. As the prostate enlarges, it can interfere with urine flow. This not only reduces the force behind the urine stream but also may prevent the bladder from completely emptying. Bladder stones and infection become more likely. While 95% of males show signs of an enlarged prostate by age seventy, less than 25% require treatment.

A nearly universal experience of aging men (women to a lesser extent) is getting up to urinate during the night. This is partly the result of the bladder not emptying completely during that last urination before bed. But this is not the whole story. In young adults, it is typical to produce greater quantities of urine in the daytime. In many elderly, this pattern is reversed. One hypothesis is that fluids trapped in legs by poor circulation are released when we become horizontal. Whatever the cause, there are obvious implications for sleep patterns—interrupted by a succession of trips to the bathroom.

Drugs or surgery are options for severe symptoms in men, but some elderly successfully reduce their nighttime interruptions with habit changes. Double voiding (a second urination shortly after the first) is worth a try, as is elevating legs before bedtime. Reducing fluid consumption and avoiding caffeine in the evenings is prudent.

For many men and women, nighttime urination becomes an "accepting the things I cannot change" situation.

Prostate cancer is the second leading cause of cancer death in men (behind lung cancer). It often causes no symptoms until it has progressed to a dangerous late stage. It is usually very slow growing as evidenced by the following statistic: Up to 30% of men have microscopic evidence of prostate cancer when they die, but the lifetime risk of dying of prostate cancer is only 3%. Thus, it is said that men are much more likely to die *with* prostate cancer than to die *of* prostate cancer.

If symptoms do develop in early stage prostate cancer, they may mimic BPH. Thus, detection can be problematic. Early diagnosis may require a biopsy, which carries the potential for damaging side effects.

61

A digital rectal exam will catch some early cancers, but not all. The PSA screening test will also detect some early cancers, but has been criticized for false positives that lead to unnecessary biopsies.

On the plus side, because prostate cancer is often slow-growing, it may never cause symptoms or threaten life. This creates the dilemma that early treatment of prostate cancer may cause more harm than "watchful waiting."

Both diagnosis and treatment of prostate cancer require an informed patient in consultation with an experienced specialist. The patient's values and desires are an essential part of the decision-making process. If a physician seems to be pushing for biopsy or surgery, a second opinion is definitely a wise course of action.

This might be a good time to reemphasize the need for caution in the selection of *all* medical professionals, treatments, and preventative strategies. Health and medicine are multibillion-dollar industries. We would like to think that health professionals and drug manufacturers are looking out for our best interest, but sadly, this is not always the case.

Avoid the latest fads for diets and nutritional supplements. Weigh side effects vs. benefits of drugs, especially those advertised in the media. (When I hear the litany of possible side effects during drug commercials, I can't believe anybody would take them!) Become well informed before submitting to any treatment or surgery. *Being a smart health consumer will save you money, safeguard your health, and possibly even save your life.*

Stiffness Is Sometimes a Good Thing

It is 1958. I am an eleven-year-old boy in the garage of my thirteen-year-old neighbor, Don. He and his friend Pete are talking together in hushed voices. I am not part of the conversation, but I clearly provide a target audience.

Don, "Did you hear what happened to Jim?"
Pete, "No. What happened?"
Don, "He was messing around with his girlfriend and
    she got mad and broke his boner."
(I can only imagine that my eyes were big as saucers at this point. They continued in serious tones.)
Don, "He went to the hospital and they put a cast on it."

Their conversation continued, but by this time, my mind had completely dissociated from my surroundings. I was imagining casts and nurses and all manner of complications. I went home in a state of complete bewilderment.

Five years later, when I had my driver's license, I resolved to educate myself more about the facts of life. (My mother and father never offered any guidance here.) I drove to our downtown public library on a mission. My heart was racing and my hands were sweaty as I looked up sexual topics in the card catalog. I did not dare ask the librarian for help. I finally located the few books that seemed relevant—in a locked glass case!

It was a long time before I learned that "boners" involved no bones. In fact, it was a long time before I learned much of anything.

****

Sexual interest is stimulated by testosterone, which naturally decreases with age (thank goodness!). While this may explain a decreased sexual appetite, it is rarely the cause of erectile dysfunction.

Half of men over sixty-five and one-quarter of men over eighty maintain full erectile function. Nearly all men have difficulty achieving an erection occasionally, but chronic difficulty may stem from several causes.

Physical factors may play a role. An erection involves the engorgement of erectile tissue in the penis with blood from the arteries. Some forms of blood vessel disease like atherosclerosis may reduce blood flow and interfere with engorgement.

Muscles at the base of the penis must contract to squeeze the veins to prevent the blood from leaving. Muscle weakness or damage can thus contribute to ED.

The entire process of erection is controlled by nerves, such that nerve damage (as may result from a prostrate biopsy) can be another physical cause of ED.

Many drugs, particularly alcohol, interfere with normal erectile function. Reduced alcohol consumption may "cure" ED.

Mental or emotional factors may play as large a role in ED as physical factors. Emotions like depression, performance anxiety, guilt, or fear may need to be addressed to achieve normal sexual performance.

Today, most cases of erectile dysfunction can be successfully treated. Depending on the professional diagnosis, both physical and emotional causes can be resolved. In addition, drugs that treat ED usually work regardless of the underlying cause. Thanks to modern pharmacology, concerns about ED are shrinking ; -)

Just don't break it.

Vaginas and Things

No personal stories to tell here. I will pass along what I have gleaned from my reading because there are many important gender-specific health issues for females.

****

Almost all Boomer women have completed *menopause*. The onset of menopause is influenced by many factors, including the age of first menstruation, the number of ovarian follicles present at birth, and the rate of loss of those follicles over the years. Generally, early menopause and the loss of fertility begin in the mid-to-late thirties. Regular menstrual cycles may continue well into the forties, but by this time natural fertility is usually quite low.

As production of hormones like estrogen, FSH, and LH change with age, menstrual cycles may become irregular, may not lead to ovulation, or may suddenly cease altogether. The typical age of menopause—defined as twelve consecutive months without a menstrual period—is usually between forty and fifty-five. The average age for menopause in U.S. women is fifty-one. The years leading up to menopause may be marked by symptoms such as hot flashes (40% of women), sleep disturbances (40%), and vaginal dryness (20%).

As hormone levels decline, the skin of the labia thins, as do the walls of the vagina. Blood flow to the vagina is significantly reduced, causing the vagina to become shorter, narrower, and drier. This may produce discomfort during intercourse. Many women continue to enjoy an active sex life after menopause, but may find supplemental lubrication helpful. Other changes include a decrease in the acidity levels in the vagina, which increases the chances of irritation and infection.

Weakening muscles may allow pelvic organs like the bladder, uterus, intestines, or rectum to shift position and push against the vagina. Weight loss and Kegel exercises help symptoms in some women. In other women, a pessary device may be inserted into the vagina for support. Extreme cases may require corrective surgery.

The reduction in the ratio between female sex hormones and testosterone following menopause increases the likelihood of hair loss or the growth of facial hair. Within five to ten years following menopause, testosterone levels drop, typically resulting in decreased sex drive.

Lack of estrogen often causes the lining of the urethra to become thin and fragile. This may lead to increased urination frequency, urgency of urination, and even uncontrollable loss of urine (urinary incontinence).

Isn't aging fun?

Whether the issue is irritation, infection, discomfort, incontinence, or sex drive, every woman should consult about the issues with her physician—preferably a gynecologist. There are effective treatments available today for almost all health concerns involving the reproductive organs.

As one example, estrogen creams may be applied to the vagina, or a ring that releases low dose estrogen may be inserted into the vagina. These steps can reduce some of the problematic effects of menopause. Because very little is absorbed into the bloodstream, this may be an appropriate measure for women who have concerns about the potential side effects of general hormone replacement therapy.

Since cancers of the breast and reproductive organs are common, it is understood that a woman should have regular cancer screenings as recommended by her doctor.

Changes in sex hormone levels in postmenopausal women also increases the risk of conditions like cardiovascular disease, stroke, osteoporosis, and Alzheimer's disease. This led to a classic case of trial and error scientific whiplash.

In an attempt to counteract the effects of menopause, estrogen replacement therapy was initiated, becoming common in the 1960s. In the peak year of 1974, 28 million prescriptions for non-birth control estrogen were written. Then a study in 1975 reported increased risk of endometrial cancer in those taking estrogen. The popularity of ERT rapidly declined.

In the 1980s, progestin was added to estrogen. This seemed to reduce the risk of endometrial cancer. Now called *Hormone Replacement Therapy* (HRT), this new regimen not only helped with the hot flashes and other side effects of menopause, it reportedly provided a protective effect against heart disease and osteoporosis.

Hints at a slightly increased risk of stroke and breast cancer did not dampen the enthusiasm for HRT in the 1990s. Then, in 2002, a large, randomized, double-blind, placebo-controlled study of 16,000 postmenopausal women was published that once again changed the prevailing wisdom about hormone therapy. The study was terminated early because of the perceived risk to study participants.

In sharp contrast to earlier studies, women taking the standard combination of estrogen and progestin (HRT) demonstrated increased risk of stroke, pulmonary embolism, and invasive breast cancer. This was especially true for women who began therapy after age sixty. Heart disease risk either increased or decreased, depending on the patient's age and other risk factors. Even though a slight decline in colorectal cancer and hip fracture was reported, the overall health risks were judged to exceed any benefit from hormone replacement therapy.

Adding to the negative press was a report in 2006 of an unexpected and rapid decline in breast cancer rates beginning in 2003—just when millions of women terminated their use of HRT. The link between these two observations is still being investigated.

What is a woman to do? This is a case where researching the latest recommendations and consulting with your physician is vital. As of this writing, the accepted guidelines are:

- Long-term use of E or E+P is not recommended, with risks generally outweighing benefits.
- Short-term use of the lowest effective dose of E or E+P may be appropriate for severe menopausal symptoms and other specific clinical applications.

Your personal history (including current age, age at menopause, genetics, and other health risk factors) and severity of menopause symptoms will greatly influence the advisability of hormone therapy. Do your homework and find a physician you trust.

Breast cancer is the most common cancer in women (excluding skin cancer). Women have an 88% chance of *never* having breast cancer, although having a close relative with breast cancer increases the risk by 2-3 times. Breast cancer risk increases with age, usually occurring in women over sixty.

As with prostate cancer in men, there is controversy about the risk of false positives screening results for breast cancer in women. Some professional organizations recommend annual mammograms beginning at age forty. Other equally esteemed organizations recommend every other year after age fifty. The decision should be made in consultation with your doctor who knows your specific risk factors.

Cancer in female reproductive organs is difficult to detect. Common examples include cancers of the ovaries, uterus, cervix, vagina, and vulva. With the exception of the Pap smear for cervical cancer, no specific screening tests are commonly used. Therefore, it is critical that women report any unusual discharge, bleeding, pressure, or pain in the pelvic area. Our basic mantra applies:

If it doesn't look right, feel right, or work right—get it checked!

Cells Gone Wild

No disease diagnosis generates more fear than the words "You have cancer." It is the second leading cause of death in the United States (only behind heart disease). To my knowledge, I have not had any form of invasive cancer, although I have had six skin cancers removed, including a potentially life-threatening melanoma.

Like most, cancer has affected people I love. A very close friend died of ovarian cancer, my mother died of melanoma, and my former wife died of brain cancer. In each case, I felt helpless in the knowledge that no treatment would provide a cure.

Today, over half of those diagnosed with cancer are alive after five years. It is our universal hope that many Baby Boomers will live to see the day when targeted treatments will substantially improve these odds.

Of course, cancer is not really a single disease. The common feature of uncontrolled cell growth links the diseases we call cancer. However, the tissue from which the cells originate defines each type of cancer and gives it unique characteristics.

If the rogue cells stay together in a defined space, the resulting tumor is called *benign* and is usually not life-threatening. If the cell growth pattern is not contained, we call it cancer. In cancer, cells *metastasize*—break away from the original tumor and spread to other locations in the body.

The odds of getting cancer increase with age. There are several factors involved. The longer a person lives, the more exposure they have to cancer-causing agents such as radiation and carcinogenic chemicals. The immune system that helps protect us against cancer becomes less efficient with age. The ability of cells to repair their own DNA damage that can lead to cancer also declines with age. For these reasons, over half of all cancer diagnosis and cancer deaths occur in people over the age of sixty-five.

Besides avoiding cancer-causing agents like sun radiation and cigarette smoke, the most effective defense against cancer is early detection. This can be difficult because the early symptoms are often vague and similar to those of other conditions. When it comes to cancer, the following acronym of warning signs reminds us to use CAUTION:

C: Change in bowel or bladder habits
A: A sore that does not heal
U: Unusual bleeding or discharge
T: Thickening or lump in breast or elsewhere
I: Indigestion or difficulty swallowing
O: Obvious change in wart or mole
N: Nagging cough or hoarseness

Enlarged lymph nodes (such as in the neck, groin or armpits), unexpected weight loss, unusual fatigue, fever, night sweats, and new or persistent pain should also be brought to a doctor's attention.

If you see a doctor and your symptoms turn out *not* to be cancer, what have you lost? It is still important to get a diagnosis and receive treatment. At the very least, you will gain peace of mind.

If it is cancer, it could save your life!

****

Our bodies are composed of nearly 100 trillion cells. On any given day, 100 billion new cells are produced to replace those that are worn out or damaged.

There are over 200 different types of tissues in the body, each being replaced at its own rate. For example, the epithelial cells that line the small intestine are replaced every 2-4 days. Skin cells are replaced every 10-30 days (producing much of the "dust" that lands on our carpets). Red blood cells last about 4 months before being recycled. Bone and muscle cells may survive 10–15 years, respectively. Some cells in the lens of the eye and the cortex of the brain last a lifetime.

DNA instructions inside the cell nucleus tightly regulate the cell division necessary for tissue renewal. Usually, the process works flawlessly, with each new cell programmed for proper growth and lifespan. But sometimes mistakes occur which produce abnormal growth and cell division. Errors in the DNA instructions can change the normal cell cycle.

Some of these DNA errors (*mutations*) are passed on through heredity. This is why certain forms of cancer are more frequent in some families. For example, a woman who inherits a defective gene called *BRCA1* has a five times greater risk of breast cancer than a woman without the gene. Over 50% of women born with a deleterious mutation in BRCA1 will develop breast cancer by age seventy. The risk of ovarian cancer in these same women may be as much as 30 times normal.

Other DNA mutations are caused by environmental factors such as radiation, cigarette smoke, and industrial chemicals. We call these factors *carcinogens*. Mutations may also result from random errors in the DNA copying process that precedes cell replication.

Since most of our DNA instructions are not involved with cell replication, most mutations are harmless. They may cause a particular cell to function abnormally, but will not produce cancer.

Everyone has inherited some mutations, and everyone has many new mutations that occur in cells during their lifespan. DNA repair mechanisms detect and fix most new mutations before they can do harm. Each strand of DNA in our cells is scanned for errors during the cell division process. If bad messages are not corrected, it often causes the cell to destroy itself. Such cell suicide is called *apoptosis*.

Our immune system is also on the lookout for potentially harmful cells. White blood cells will engulf and digest body cells that are not operating normally.

As you can see, the body has several layers of protection against the development of cancer. Cancer requires a sequence of mistakes and failures that fortunately is very rare for any particular cell. Even with the tremendous number of cells in the body, *over 60% of all people will never be diagnosed with any form of cancer in their lifetime. As of this writing, approximately 80% of men and 86% of women will **not** die from it.*

Cancer is complex. In the most general terms, cancer is a failure of the genes that regulate cell growth and reproduction. It usually requires the alteration of many genes in a cell. Here is an outline of the process.

Two general categories of genes are involved in the development of cancer—*oncogenes* and *tumor suppressor genes.* Normal oncogenes promote cell growth and cell division. Normal tumor suppressor genes inhibit cell division and limit cell survival. (BRCA1 is a tumor suppressor gene.)

Typically, cancer cannot develop without the combined changes to several oncogenes and tumor suppressor genes within a particular cell. In other words, genes that normally promote cell growth and division become overactive and genes that normally suppress cell division become underactive.

Mutations in oncogenes and tumor suppressor genes have long been the foundation of our understanding of cancer genesis. Increasingly, researchers have found that changes in the genes that *regulate* oncogenes and tumor suppressor genes play a critical role. A change in a regulator gene is called an *epigenetic* alteration.

Whether the mutation is in the gene itself or in its regulator, a cell that starts out as a dutiful and compliant member of cell society goes wild—dividing out of control and crowding the normal cells until those cells cannot do their job. This is cancer.

For example, let's say that a particular form of lung cancer is triggered by changes to three oncogenes and two tumor suppressor genes. (5 total)

(1) By random chance, Tom is born with one damaged oncogene inherited from his mom. This mutation would be found in all of his body cells.

(2) Tom grows up in Southern California in the years before air pollution controls are implemented. On his school playground during a severe smog episode, a chemical in the air triggers a mutation in another oncogene in one of his lung cells. Undetected by his immune system, this mutation is passed to all the decedents of this cell.

(3) Tom's father smokes in the car with the windows closed, so a regulator of a tumor suppressor gene (in the already altered lung cell) is damaged by second-hand smoke. Thus, before Tom enters high school, he is more than halfway to developing lung cancer.

(4) During college, Tom begins smoking and develops a nicotine addiction that he cannot overcome until he is middle aged. During those years, carcinogens in the cigarette smoke mutate an oncogene regulator.

For the next forty years, any mutations in the pre-cancerous lung cells are caught and corrected by DNA repair mechanisms. Other potential cancer cells spontaneously undergo apoptosis or are destroyed by the immune system. Tom stays healthy.

(5) Finally, just after his sixtieth birthday, an error during cell division mutates the last tumor suppressor gene. This sends the lung cell into uncontrolled cell division. His aging immune system does not stop the growth. The initial symptoms of chronic coughing and shortness of breath he attributes to allergies and old age. By the time Tom has serious symptoms and sees a doctor, his disease is terminal.

This example is not a scientific explanation of the development of lung cancer. It is only designed to show how cancer can be the result of cumulative effects of heredity, exposure to carcinogens, and errors in DNA replication. We cannot change our heredity, but we can reduce our exposure to cancer risk factors, get cancer screenings when appropriate, and be aware of cancer warning signs.

Currently, over 25% of cancer deaths are caused by tobacco. This number will decline as fewer people are exposed to cigarette smoke.

Another 30% of cancer deaths are attributed to overweight and poor nutrition—a percentage that unfortunately may rise with the obesity epidemic.

Nearly 20% of cancer deaths may be triggered by viral diseases. (When certain viruses invade cells, they cause DNA mutations. Hepatitis and human papillomavirus are examples.)

Radiation is responsible for another 10%.

Less than 10% of cancers have a strictly genetic basis.

Obviously, the first step in avoiding cancer death is avoiding carcinogens in our personal environment. Nevertheless, no matter how careful one is, the risk of cancer will never be zero.

I want to emphasize that we Boomers have a 60% chance of never having cancer and less than 50% chance of dying from it if we are diagnosed. **Cancer is not an automatic death sentence. The key is early detection and treatment.**

By this stage in our lives, most of us have known someone who died of cancer. Often, they might have been cured if the cancer had been found earlier. As tragic as this is, it is even more tragic if we do not learn from it.

Stay in tune with your body—notice when things change—and don't swim in that Egyptian river.

How Sweet It Is – Not

Diabetes is common in older people, although 75% of us will manage to avoid this disease. It is diagnosed as high levels of glucose (sugar) in the blood (*hyperglycemia*). Diabetes is the result of deficiencies in insulin production or utilization. (Insulin helps transport sugar into body cells from the blood.) My father-in-law died of diabetes. Before his death, he suffered the loss of both legs through amputation.

Such heartbreaking complications are common. Diabetes damages blood vessels, particularly the tiny capillaries. Narrowing of and leakage from these vessels interferes with blood flow to the tissues. This can lead to heart disease, stroke, kidney failure, blindness, loss of sensation in extremities, and amputation.

The initial symptoms of diabetes are often excessive urination and abnormal thirst. This is because the body is trying to excrete the excess sugar in the blood that cannot enter the cells of the body. **Increased hunger and unexpected weight loss are also symptoms**. This is because the body cannot access the energy-rich sugar in the blood made available by the digestive system.

The good news is that diabetes often can be prevented. The main risk factor is obesity. Changes in weight, diet, and exercise can dramatically lower risk.

If diabetes does develop, it may be well controlled through a variety of treatment options including diet restrictions, medications, and insulin replacement.

****

After a meal or snack, sugar is absorbed into the bloodstream from the digestive system. The pancreas responds by producing insulin that also enters the blood stream. Insulin helps move sugar across cell membranes into body cells where it can be utilized for cell energy. If the body cannot produce or properly respond to insulin, the result is diabetes (*diabetes mellitus*).

There are two forms of diabetes. In *type 1* diabetes, the body's immune system destroys the pancreas cells that produce insulin. Symptoms of hyperglycemia usually show up in childhood or young adulthood. As of now, this form of diabetes cannot be prevented. Lifelong management, including insulin supplementation, can significantly reduce the serious complications.

Over 90% of diabetes is labeled *type 2*. In this case, the pancreas produces enough insulin, but body cells do not respond properly to it. This condition is called *insulin resistance*. In order to transport glucose into body cells, insulin must combine with receptors on the surface of cells. In the case of type 2 diabetes, the insulin receptors are modified or reduced in number. This prevents insulin from completing its mission.

Age and heredity play a role. If both of your parents had diabetes, your risk rises to 50%. But by far the main risk factor for diabetes is obesity. More than 80% of type 2 diabetics are overweight when they develop the disease.

In a major study by the National Institute of Health over a 3-year period, *modifying diet and exercise to produce a 15 lb weight loss reduced diabetes risk by 58% (71% in those over age sixty).*

As a normal part of aging, insulin production decreases and insulin resistance increases. This, however, does not usually lead to diabetes. Eating too much and exercising too little are the basic causes of type 2 diabetes.

Recent studies suggest that eating foods high in sugar and carbohydrate (corn syrup, white bread, white rice) produces spikes in blood sugar, sometimes referred to as glycemic stress. This may increase the risk of diabetes (as well as heart disease and macular degeneration). These are long-term consequences of dietary habits, not the result of occasional indulgence.

Being proactive in lifestyle choices can lead to sweet results!

The Ailment-ary Canal

In my thirty-four years as a teacher, I occasionally battled digestive issues. I think I had a mild form of *irritable bowel syndrome* (IBS). It was sometimes uncomfortable, but not debilitating. I also had episodes of abdominal pain and fever, diagnosed as *diverticulitis*. My gastroenterologist warned me I might have to have a bad section of my intestine removed (as had happened to my father). Fortunately, modified eating habits and antibiotics always cleared up my outbreaks, and it never came to that.

When I retired from teaching, my digestive issues miraculously disappeared (unless I overindulge).

I did have one digestive issue that led to surgery. It all started at a Dodgers baseball game. More specifically, it started with a Dodger Dog—or several of them. The night after the game, I awakened to excruciating abdominal pain. It was the worst I had ever felt. (Kidney stones came years later.) I could not sleep and contemplated going to the emergency room. I toughed it out, and the pain subsided slightly toward morning. I saw the doctor the next day. Tests revealed *gallstones*.

I was sent to a surgeon who offered me an interesting choice. I could have the surgery immediately using the old-fashioned method of a major abdominal incision and weeks of recovery. Or, if I could wait, the doctor would complete his training in laparoscopic surgery—which would only require three tiny incisions and a week's recovery. I opted for door number two.

The doctor explained that the gallbladder stores bile produced by the liver. It releases bile to help digest fats. The stones (deposits) in my bile duct were causing pain during gall bladder contractions—like when I tried to digest the Dodger Dogs.

I went on a completely non-fat diet for three months until the doctor said he was ready. I was grateful to be one of his first patients to receive the new procedure.

As with all body systems, aging affects digestive tract functions. In most people, these changes are less noticeable than are those to vision, hair, or skin—but they are just as common.

Muscles of the esophagus contract less forcefully, sometimes creating swallowing problems. (I notice I sometimes have trouble with large pills.) The stomach holds less food than it used to because it is less elastic. (No more sixteen pancake breakfasts!) The stomach also empties more slowly. (Five o'clock dinners are a senior joke—with practical benefits for digestion before bedtime.)

Another common digestive issue is *Gastroesophageal Reflux Disease (GERD)*, also known as acid reflux. Caused by weakness or relaxation of the sphincter at the top of the stomach, it allows acid to back up into the esophagus. Symptoms include heartburn, regurgitation, sore throat, chest pain, and coughing. Some find relief with dietary changes and over the counter medications. If this is not sufficient, it is vital to get medical treatment. Chronic GERD can lead to esophageal damage and even cancer. Don't just "live with it." Physicians have effective treatments.

Older folks typically eat less. The production of hormones that stimulate appetite is reduced with age. Food may also be less appetizing as the ability to taste and smell decline. (Some may find they use more sugar, salt, or spices to compensate.)

The production of digestive enzymes declines with age. A reduction in lactase, for example, may produce difficulty digesting dairy products—*lactose intolerance.* Bloating and diarrhea after drinking milk are clues.

The slowed movement of waste through the large intestine may contribute to constipation. Getting enough fiber and fluids becomes imperative.

A young digestive system usually adjusts to the recklessness of poor diet and overconsumption. Such is not the case as we age. Good choices and moderation may cure many digestive ailments.

****

Diverticulosis is the formation of pouches (*diverticula*) along the inside wall of the digestive track. They can occur anywhere from the esophagus to the rectum, but usually form in the large intestine. About 40% of the risk is genetic, but a highly refined, low-fiber diet contributes. Contrary to common mythology, there is no evidence that eating nuts or seeds contributes to its development.

Diverticula can range in diameter from 3 mm to 3 cm. Seventy percent of us will be free of diverticula at the age of fifty, but the incidence increases steadily with age.

Eighty percent of those who *do* develop diverticulosis have no serious issues with it. In some people, however, the pouches become infected by bacteria and cause a disease called *diverticulitis*.

Symptoms of diverticulitis include pain (usually in the lower left abdominal quadrant), fever, and increased white blood cell count. Treatment may be as simple as a low residue diet to give the colon rest. Antibiotics are given in some cases, but their routine use is not supported.

Irritable bowel syndrome is characterized by abdominal pain and bloating. Alteration of bowel habits may range from constipation to extreme diarrhea. The most accepted theory is that IBS stems from a disorder in the communication between the brain and gastrointestinal tract. Irritations such as stress, infections, or overeating may trigger episodes.

If testing reveals no organic disease responsible for symptoms, then psychological intervention, dietary adjustment, or medications may be involved in treatment.

Bile is secreted by the liver to aid in emulsifying fats. This breaks fat into smaller droplets that can be more effectively digested. Bile is temporarily stored in the gall bladder, then released into the digestive tract following a meal. While the bile is stored, *gallstones* sometimes form as precipitates of cholesterol, bilirubin, or other components of bile.

If these hardened deposits lodge in the bile duct, they may cause intensifying pain in the upper right portion of the abdomen. The pain may last from minutes to hours.

Several factors increase the risk of gallstones, including being older, being female, being overweight, and having a family history. Fortunately, over 70% of us will not experience gallstones by age seventy-five.

You do not need a gallbladder to live. If it is surgically removed, the bile flows directly from the liver into the digestive tract. Some patients report digestive issues (like occasional diarrhea) after removal, but most notice no differences from before surgery—except the absence of pain!

Colorectal cancer is the second most deadly. It usually has no symptoms until it is life threatening. Colonoscopy screening should begin at age fifty (forty-five for African Americans). New, less intrusive tests are being developed and may be discussed with your doctor. In the meantime, do not avoid colonoscopy. It can be a life or death decision.

Childbirth for Men

If you have ever had a kidney stone, you probably have a story to tell. Here is mine.

Of course, it had to strike while I was teaching. I was in the middle of an AP Biology class when I started to feel the pain. It felt a little like an urgent bladder call, but seemed to go up my back on the lower right side. At first, I thought I could wait to deal with it on my lunch break, but the intensity grew quickly. My class was full of super responsible kids, so I finally excused myself and made a quick trip to the restroom. When I began to urinate, I was completely shocked. Blood.

I knew this was not good. I asked a colleague to cover my class, told the office what was going on, and drove the short distance to my house. By this time, I was in excruciating pain. My wife met me at the door.

"Drive me to the emergency room," I said. It was difficult to talk, but I gave her the short version of the story as we drove. I opened the window. I felt like throwing up.

"I might pass out. Just get me there," I said. The pain was more intense than anything I had ever felt. I really did think I might pass out. I implored her to run a red light, but she was smart enough to ignore my plea.

I was relieved to be in the emergency room—until everything went into slow motion.

"Can I see a doctor *now*?" I was almost crying.

"I need to get some information," the receptionist replied. "We will get you in as soon as possible."

I registered in agony. She told me to have a seat in the waiting room. The pain was off the chart.

Finally, I couldn't stand it and returned to the receptionist.

"Can I just have something for the pain," I pleaded.

"It might interfere with your diagnosis. We can't give you anything until we know what is going on," she answered. Her voice did not seem all that sympathetic. I hoped she got a kidney stone some day.

I felt like I had to urinate again, so I went to the restroom. When I returned to my seat, I noticed the pain became slightly less intense—perhaps dropping from eleven to nine on the ten-point pain scale.

When I finally saw the doctor, he seemed disappointed that my pain was subsiding. He was hoping to get a sample of the stone for analysis. Their composition can hold a clue to prevention. He speculated that I had passed the stone in the restroom. He must have been right because I urinated into a strainer for a week and there was no sign of a stone.

My wife said that now I knew what childbirth felt like. If that is true, I am surprised we have a population problem.

****

Kidney stones are solid masses that form from minerals in the urine. Most are based around calcium. They may range from a grain of sand size to pearl size. If they reach about 3 mm in diameter, they can block the *ureter* (urine tube from the kidney). This is the source of the debilitating symptoms of pain, nausea, vomiting, and sometimes bleeding.

Pain control is the primary treatment. Most cases resolve themselves in hours to days. Hospital procedures are necessary in stubborn cases.

People who have experienced a kidney stone or have a family history are advised to limit intake of animal proteins, salt, and sugar. Calcium intake should be moderated, and large doses of vitamin C supplements avoided. Cola soft drinks, overweight, and certain drugs may also play a role.

By far the most important recommendation for prevention of kidney stones is avoiding dehydration. Water intake will vary depending on exercise, weather, food intake, body size, etc. The oft-heard "rule" of drinking 8 eight-ounce glasses of fluid (mostly water) a day is a good starting approximation. Properly hydrated, you are rarely thirsty, you have light colored urine, and you produce six or more cups of urine a day.

Mercifully, over 90% of the U.S. population will miss the "opportunity" to experience a kidney stone.

Kidney and urinary tract disorders may be of serious concern in some elderly. Kidney function gradually decreases after age thirty, but even those above age eighty typically maintain over 50% of their original capabilities. This is usually sufficient to prevent any threat to wellbeing. However, seniors may be less able to cope optimally with either dehydration or excess water intake.

The elderly are also more susceptible to kidney disease. For example, older kidneys become more vulnerable to drug toxicity. Because 20% of blood coming from the heart passes through the kidneys, drugs tend to become concentrated there. Also, liver enzymes that normally break down drugs are reduced with age, leaving more toxic drugs in the blood.

Despite all of the jokes (and depressing TV ads), *incontinence* is *not* an inevitable part of aging. Between seventy and ninety percent of older people report full bladder control, although that number drops to fifty percent in those who are institutionalized.

Two major causes of incontinence are weakened muscle tissue (common in postmenopausal women when estrogen levels decline) and increased urine retention (common in men with decreased urine flow due to enlarged prostate).

Weight loss can provide positive improvement in bladder control, especially in women. Kegel exercises to strengthen the pelvic floor muscles and urinary sphincter muscles may also be effective. In one study, women who lost weight and exercised reduced their incidence of incontinence by over 70%.

Men who receive treatment for their BPH may reduce their incidence of incontinence since the bladder can empty more completely.

For both men and women, several medical interventions can be effective in treating incontinence. The choice will depend on the individual's symptoms, health history, and physical condition.

A Stroke of Bad Luck

A neighbor of ours suffered a stroke last year. (If you live in a 55+ community, you know someone who has suffered almost every imaginable malady.) Thanks to quick treatment, rehab, and the healing of time, you would never suspect it today. We have learned much about recovery from this potentially debilitating event.

A stroke is damage to a portion of the brain caused by an interruption in the supply of blood. The results of stroke depend on what part of the brain is damaged. Effects can include muscle weakness or paralysis, coordination issues, vision or hearing loss, and speech problems. Since each hemisphere of the brain controls the opposite side of the body, the effects are usually limited to one side.

Early treatment is vital to the long-term outcome. Knowing the symptoms of stroke is imperative. ***Any of the following should trigger an immediate call to 911.***

- Face drooping. The inability to make a symmetrical smile is a good test.
- Sudden difficulty moving or abnormal sensations in the extremities. Arm weakness is a good test.
- Sudden difficulty speaking or understanding.
- Sudden changes in vision.
- Sudden dizziness or loss of balance.
- Sudden severe headache.

It used to be thought that the brain could not heal—that any brain damage was permanent. Today we know that brain functions can be shifted to different areas, new connections can form, and in some cases, new nerve cells may actually grow. With the proper treatment and rehabilitation, the brain has remarkable "plasticity." It is vital that the stroke victim takes rehab seriously and put in the effort to maximize recovery.

That being said, the damage from stroke can be life threatening. Stroke is the third leading cause of death in the U.S., accounting for 5% of all mortality.

Risk factors for stroke mirror those for heart disease (high cholesterol levels, atherosclerosis, high blood pressure, diabetes, obesity, inactivity, etc.). Once again, lifestyle choices are the primary determinant of risk.

Some heart disorders such as valve problems and arrhythmias increase the risk of blood clots that can cause a stroke. Blood thinners may be prescribed in such cases.

****

There are two types of stroke. *Hemorrhagic stroke* is caused by a broken blood vessel in the brain. Weak vessels or unusually high pressure are typically to blame. The resulting bleed not only interferes with blood supply but also creates swelling that can damage brain tissue.

Eighty-five percent of strokes are labeled *ischemic*. This kind of stroke is caused by a blockage in a brain blood vessel, usually by a blood clot. *It is critical that clot-busting drugs be administered within 3 hours of symptoms to minimize damage.*

A *transient ischemic attack* (TIA) causes symptoms similar to a stroke but usually lasts less than 90 minutes. Immediate medical attention is still critical because a TIA is often a warning sign of an impending stroke.

Brain Fade

I mentioned before that the most feared diagnosis is cancer. Perhaps equally feared would be a diagnosis of Alzheimer's or some other form of dementia. In cancer, the primary fear is of pain, physical degradation, and death. In dementia, the fear is of memory loss, mental degradation, and death. I would not want to choose between the two.

Not remembering as well as we once did (*benign forgetfulness*) is a nearly universal complaint in older adults. When my wife or I cannot remember someone's name or come up with the right vocabulary word, we laugh about having a "brain burp." We also can still make fun of having "old-timers' disease" when we can't remember if we have seen a particular movie. Beneath the laughter, the fear of brain function decline is very real. After all, the brain holds our memories—and our very identity.

Even in healthy aging, the brain undergoes changes. Certain areas shrink and communications between neurons (nerve cells) slow. Blood flow is reduced as arteries and capillaries become less efficient. Modest declines in the ability to learn new things and retrieve information are normal. Yet *given enough time*, many in their seventies and eighties perform these mental tasks as well as young adults. *Major cognitive decline is not inevitable as people age.*

There are several forms of dementia. Alzheimer's is the most well known. In keeping with our positive approach, the following chart shows the chances of NOT having dementia as we age.

Age	No Alzheimer's	No Dementia (any kind)
71-79	97.7%	95%
80-89	82%	76%
90+	70%	63%

Scientists talk about *cognitive reserve*—the ability of the brain to adapt to the physical changes of aging and continue to operate effectively. Genetics, education, and lifestyle support the development of cognitive reserve. **The active process of learning increases the number of brain cells, increases connections between brain cells, increases the number of glial (neuron support) cells, and improves blood flow to the brain.**

In addition to continued learning, regular exercise greatly benefits brain health. Controlling weight, blood pressure, and cholesterol is helpful, as is a healthy diet with plenty of fruits and vegetables. Maintaining close social ties with family, friends, and community is also beneficial.

The phrase *use it or lose it* applies to brain health. Studies have shown that cognitive training exercises for processing speed, reasoning, and memory can counteract the degree of decline normally expected in the elderly for periods of fourteen years and longer. Select activities, hobbies, and mental exercises that keep your brain sharp.

****

One of the hallmarks of an unhealthy brain is *confusion*—the failure to process information correctly. This may manifest as the inability to follow a conversation, answer questions appropriately, pay attention, keep track of information, or remember things.

If confusion develops suddenly (hours to days) and is limited in duration (days to weeks), it may be categorized as *delirium*. The manifestations of delirium may vary depending on environmental factors such as fatigue and time of day. It is usually caused by conditions such as infection, dehydration, stress, a side effect of medication, or withdrawal from medication.

People who display the sudden onset of delirium require immediate medical attention. Treatment will often return normal function. Despite the symptoms of confusion and memory loss, delirium is not a step on the way to dementia.

Confusion that develops slowly (months to years) is usually caused by a chronic brain disorder and is referred to as *dementia*. When dementia first develops, it has less to do with the ability to pay attention (like delirium) and more to do with memory loss. However, all aspects of brain function slowly and steadily deteriorate. This robs people of the ability to think, remember, communicate, and control behavior. (The old fashioned word was *senility*.)

There are several forms of dementia produced by different brain changes. Vascular dementia is caused by strokes. Lewy body dementia is associated with Parkinson's disease. Other forms are caused by hydrocephalus (increased brain fluid).

By far, the most common form of dementia is *Alzheimer's disease*. At this point, it is a progressive, incurable disease that eventually ends in death. The exact cause of Alzheimer's is unknown, but there is a clear hereditary component. The disease is characterized by low levels of acetylcholine in the brain. This neurotransmitter helps nerve cells communicate with each other. The brains of Alzheimer's patients also have an abundance of "plaques" and "tangles"—forms of misfolded proteins.

The symptoms of Alzheimer's disease are similar to other forms of dementia. They include memory loss, language problems, personality changes, disruptive behaviors, and difficulty with daily activities. In most people, the first sign of Alzheimer's is the forgetting of recent events. Progression is unpredictable, but people generally live 8-10 years after diagnosis.

Currently, treatments for Alzheimer's and other forms of dementia may temporarily slow decline, but not cure the disease. Research breakthroughs hold out the promise that this may change in our lifetime.

Forgetfulness is not always a sign of dementia. Some people have slight problems remembering things and show minimal declines in other brain functions. This condition is called *age-related cognitive impairment*. It does not steadily progress and does not affect normal functioning in the world.

Other older people become very forgetful. This is called *mild cognitive impairment* or *benign senescent forgetfulness*. For about half of those with this condition, dementia never develops. For the other half, Alzheimer's disease will slowly develop over the next 3-5 years.

Parkinson's disease is not a form of dementia, but I included it here because it is a form of progressive nerve degeneration. Specifically, the basal ganglia of the cerebrum deteriorate, producing less of the neurotransmitter dopamine. As a result, smooth coordination of muscle movement is compromised. Also, the imbalance between dopamine and acetylcholine neurotransmitters produces the characteristic tremor.

Typically, the symptoms of Parkinson's disease begin subtly with tremors of the hands while at rest. A gradual progression over years may eventually interfere with walking and the completion of daily activities.

No treatment can cure Parkinson's or stop its progression. Some drugs, however, may effectively control symptoms for many years.

Perchance to Dream

With some envy, my wife claims that I am asleep before my head hits the pillow. I have always been a good sleeper. I tell my wife that it is because I have a guilt-free conscience.

The two main sleep disturbances of aging are *insomnia* and excessive daytime sleepiness. Although common and natural, poor sleep habits may contribute to both.

Insomnia may include difficulty in getting to sleep, awakening early, or interrupted sleep. Thankfully, about 60% of older folks report no insomnia.

Some elderly sleep is disturbed by leg twitches or discomfort. Leg muscle contractions can be caused by a loss of coordination between excitatory and inhibitory motor nerves. Arthritis and other sources of pain can also awaken individuals. We have already discussed how the need for nighttime urination may interrupt sleep.

Often, older people tend to go to bed earlier, take longer to get to sleep, and wake up earlier than they did when they were younger. Also, they spend less time in the deeper, most restful stages of sleep. As a result, they may feel less rested and alert when they awaken. They may also be more prone to napping during the day as the body tries to "catch up" after a poor night's sleep.

****

Insomnia may be a symptom of a long list of physical problems including osteoarthritis, gastroesophageal reflux, BPH, and heart disease. Psychological problems ranging from anxiety to depression may also interfere with sleep. Treating the underlying cause is the best first step toward improvement.

Changing personal habits can also help. Following is a list of behaviors that have proven valuable in the quest for a good night's sleep:

- Get regular daytime exercise and exposure to sunlight. (Avoid exercise in the evenings.)
- Eat the last meal at least 3 hours before bedtime.
- Avoid drugs that disturb sleep—like caffeine and decongestants—especially after lunch.
- Avoid alcohol in the evening and excessive drinking anytime.
- Have a consistent bedtime and bedtime rituals.
- Maintain a dark, cool, quiet environment. (Electronic divices including TV, tablets, or phones may seem relaxing, but they can stimulate the brain in ways that interfere with sleep. Try "no screens in the bedroom" for a while and see if it helps.)
- Avoid daytime napping, or if necessary, limit naps to less than half an hour. (Older people tend to nap more than younger people because they are less stimulated and less physically active.)

Changing habits is challenging, but vastly superior to reliance on chemical sleep aids.

Sleep apnea is a temporary interruption in breathing caused by the partial or complete obstruction of the airway that occurs repeatedly during sleep. Sleep apnea usually causes episodes of loud snoring and breathing cessation followed by gasping, shortness of breath, and restlessness.

Most people who snore do not have sleep apnea. However, it is very important to be diagnosed because sleep apnea lowers blood oxygen levels and can have serious side effects. In addition to being irritable and poorly rested, people with sleep apnea are at increased risk for high blood pressure, stroke, heart attack, confusion, and depression.

Those with airways that are naturally narrow—or are narrowed by fat deposits from obesity—are prone to sleep apnea. Alcohol and certain sleep aids that relax throat muscles may also add to the risk.

Fortunately, sleep apnea can usually be effectively treated. Those who have corrected their sleep apnea are universally grateful for the change it makes in their lives.

Stress: Friend and Foe

Stress has always been part of human existence. As an animal with limited speed and few defenses, our survival in the natural world was always tenuous. Our prehistoric ancestors were most likely to die at the claws of an animal predator—or the hands of a human competitor.

Today, most humans will die in a completely different way—slow deterioration caused by, or accelerated by, stress. Stress is the body's reaction to stressors. A *stressor* is any event that disrupts homeostasis (the body's natural balance). In psychological terms, a stressor is a real or perceived threat to our physical, emotional, or social well-being.

You have probably heard of the *fight or flight response.* Evolution has provided us with this stress response to deal with emergencies, as when a lion chased us across the savannah. Under such conditions, the sympathetic nervous system releases epinephrine and norepinephrine (also called adrenaline and noradrenaline) which place the body in survival mode. Heartbeat, blood pressure, breathing, and muscle tension increase in preparation for action. Nonessential functions like those of the digestive system and immune system are inhibited.

Our fight or flight mechanisms are designed to last minutes, the length of a typical emergency situation. Our brain, however, treats psychological threats the same as it treats an encounter with a predator. The same fight or flight response that allowed our ancestors to survive a dreaded lion is now triggered by thoughts of our dreaded boss as we drive to work.

93

This means that living in our modern world of multitasking, deadlines, and high volume social interaction can lead to chronic stress. Such stress puts our body in constant survival mode. It is easy to understand why unrelenting stress reactions lead to digestive issues, heart disease, and immune system compromise. The mechanisms designed for short-term survival now cause long-term damage.

I have already mentioned several stress-related medical issues from my life. During my teaching career, I suffered digestive problems, heart palpitations, and sinus infections on a regular basis. Since my retirement, I have experienced dramatic improvement in all of these areas. My own experience has led me to become a true believer in the adverse effects of stress on health.

I have also seen the serious impact of stress in my family. When my brother was killed by a drunk driver, my mother never fully recovered emotionally—and was dead herself within two years. Unfortunately, these kinds of anecdotes are common.

Chronic stress is clearly harmful. Unexpectedly, however, moderate stress of short duration has been shown to provide positive benefits. Most notably, it can strengthen our immune system, improve brain function, and keep our body fit (by properly stressing muscles).

The goal, therefore, is not to live a stress-free life. The goal is to learn to manage our stress to keep it from becoming chronic and harmful. As is often true, balance is the key. Physical and emotional stress does not have to threaten our health as long as we balance it with times of relaxation and calmness.

To this end, each of us must find activities that give us periods of stress relief. For some, it may be as simple as a daily walk. For others, it may be meditation or yoga. Immersing ourselves in enjoyable hobbies like reading, art, music, crafts, or woodworking can provide similar benefits. The key is to set aside the time each day.

****

In addition to epinephrine and norepinephrine (which act in seconds), a longer lasting class of hormones called *glucocorticoids* sustains the stress response. These are pro-inflammatory chemicals whose long-term presence can damage the body in several ways:

- Elevated levels of glucocorticoids (like cortisol) affect brain neurons, interfering with learning and memory while increasing anxiety.
- If we are constantly mobilizing energy, we do not store surplus energy, causing us to fatigue more rapidly. We even run a higher risk of developing diabetes.
- Chronically elevated blood pressure damages the interiors of blood vessels and strains the heart.
- Repair of bones and other tissues is interrupted when our stress reaction reallocates resources.
- Chronic or repeated stress response can suppress the immune system, making us more susceptible to disease or making disease recovery more difficult.

These negative effects of stress are not automatic, but as is often the case, they interact with natural human variations. The most accurate thing we can say is that chronic stress increases our *chances* of these negative health consequences.

In one classic study of stress and heart disease, monkeys were allowed to form social groups until normal dominance hierarchies were established. Subordinate monkeys at the bottom of the hierarchy—who have little control of their social environment and few outlets when stressful events occur—were much more likely to develop atherosclerotic plaques in their arteries.

The same occurred in other groups of monkeys where the dominance system was unstable (with the frequent addition and subtraction of group members). In fact, monkeys who were struggling to maintain their position at the top of the ever-shifting hierarchy were much more likely to suffer heart attacks. In both studies, there was a direct correlation between social stress and artery plaque formation.

Stimulation of the sympathetic nervous system during stress has two contrasting effects on the digestive system. When the lion is chasing you, energy comes from immediate supplies in the muscles and liver. Digestion is not a priority, so peristalsis of the stomach and small intestines stops. Meanwhile, all of the waste in the large intestines is just dead weight, so contractions in the large intestines accelerate in an attempt to jettison the excess baggage. This is why gastrointestinal diseases like colitis and irritable bowel syndrome are the most common disorders resulting from chronic stress.

I could continue to chronicle the effects of stress from ulcers to memory loss, but I think you get the picture. The stress response is a positive adaptation to emergencies, but when the body pumps out stress hormones too often or too long, they damage health.

(If you want more details, Stanford Professor of Biology and Neuroscience Robert Sapolsky has written a highly informative and readable book on the subject called *Why Zebras Don't Get Ulcers.*)

Down but Not Out

At some point after my "domino" series of heath challenges, I hit a low point. My doctor had put me on Coumadin for fear that another bout of atrial fibrillation would cause a stroke. This required frequent blood tests—which made me feel like a permanent patient. My physical conditioning was at an all time low such that even a short walk felt like a major effort. My episodes of afib had reawakened deep fears from childhood that my heart might fail. Added to this were the terrifying memories of suffocation I experienced during my pulmonary embolism. I found myself in a constant state of anxiety.

I was not seriously suicidal, but I admit that I wondered how many Vicodin (left from my Achilles surgery) it would take to end my constant discomfort. Life in my current state did not seem worth living.

Looking back, I think I had fallen into a mild depression. I have newfound understanding and respect for those that suffer from this debilitating condition. Because my depression was not severe, the passage of time and some positive health choices helped me work my way back.

I told my doctor that I wanted to get off the Coumadin. He agreed to support my decision on two conditions:

1)   Genetic testing had to show that I did not have an abnormal tendency toward blood clots.

2)   I experienced no episodes of afib for six months.

I met both of those conditions. Once off the Coumadin, my anxiety about ill health improved.

The other thing I did was to become more physically active. I restarted my pattern of doing yoga stretches in the morning. I alternated days of strength training and cardiovascular workouts at the gym. Once my conditioning improved, I started playing pickleball again. The enjoyment of the game and spending time with friends completed my return to being "myself" again.

****

Depression is defined as an extraordinary sadness that interferes with the ability to function. It is not a sign of weakness or a character flaw, but a medical condition. You would be just as wrong to say, "Snap out of your depression," to someone as you would be to say, "Snap out of your diabetes." People who suffer depression do not need cheering up. They need our compassion and support, but most of all they need *medical treatment*.

The National Institute of Mental Health lists the following as signs of depression if they persist for more than a couple of weeks:

- Persistent sad, anxious, or "empty" mood
- Feelings of hopelessness, pessimism
- Feelings of guilt, worthlessness, helplessness
- Loss of interest or pleasure in hobbies, activities
- Decreased energy, fatigue, being "slowed down"
- Difficulty concentrating, remembering, making decisions
- Difficulty sleeping, awakening early or late
- Appetite and/or weight changes
- Thoughts of death or suicide

Clearly, these may be symptoms of other problems, particularly in seniors. Some medications have these side effects. Some physical problems such as vascular changes in the brain or thyroid malfunctions may cause them. The important point is to seek evaluation by a physician to start the healing process. If it is depression, even the most severe cases can be treated.

Fifteen million Americans have depression. Having one parent with a mood disorder nearly triples the risk, and having two effected parents increases the risk five-fold. Over 40,000 commit suicide each year in the U.S.

Physical factors play a role in depression, including genetics, hormone imbalance, brain structure, and brain chemistry. Life events such as trauma, abuse, loss, and other stressors may trigger or contribute to the development of depression.

Seniors may be particularly vulnerable. We face the health challenges of aging. We may experience the loss of purpose and identity that can accompany retirement. We grieve the loss of loved ones. We may end up living alone or in an institution. We contemplate our own mortality.

It is estimated that 15-20% of Americans over the age of sixty-five struggle with at least one episode of serious depression. Suicide is the tenth leading cause of death in the U.S. Historically, seniors have the highest suicide rates of any age group. The suffering can be limited and the disease treated if we reach out for professional help. A primary care physician can begin the process and refer us to other professionals as necessary.

For immediate help, call the confidential 24hr National Suicide Prevention Lifeline at 1-800-273-TALK (8255) or go online at www.suicidepreventionlifeline.org.

Anxiety is worry and intense nervousness that interferes with the ability to function. It may accompany many physical disorders and can be a side effect of medications. It is less common than depression in the elderly. Less than 4% of us will be diagnosed with a general anxiety disorder (defined as at least six months of unrelenting fear and nervousness).

Other anxiety disorders include obsessive-compulsive disorder, phobias, post-traumatic stress disorder, and panic disorder. These conditions usually respond well to a combination of medication and psychotherapy.

Alcohol is not a medication, yet some turn to it to solve problems, including depression and anxiety. More seniors are hospitalized for alcohol-related problems than for heart attacks.

The aging body processes alcohol differently, producing greater negative effects. Alcohol interacts with medications to produce side effects such as balance issues (leading to hip fractures), bleeding (with NSAIDs), and liver damage (with acetaminophen).

Heavy drinking may worsen urinary incontinence, depression, sleep disturbances, memory loss, dementia, high blood pressure, and nutritional deficiencies. Also, regularly consuming more than two drinks a day has been linked to certain cancers and liver disorders.

One in five Boomers has a substance abuse problem. Acknowledgment is the first step toward recovery, freedom, and health. Treatment options are available in nearly every community. (Search online for Substance Abuse Treatment Centers, Alcoholics Anonymous, Narcotics Anonymous, Al-Anon, etc.)

Depression, anxiety, and substance abuse are issues where we can support our fellow Boomers. Be a true friend and start the conversation.

The Rollercoaster

Health in the aging adult can be like a rollercoaster ride. We are at a high point of health and vitality when suddenly everything falls out from under us. It could be a cancer diagnosis, a heart problem, pneumonia, or a broken hip. The ups and downs of illness can leave our confidence shaken, reminding us that we are aging—and eventually mortal.

The amusement ride analogy is insightful in another way. Like an old-fashioned rollercoaster, we may never quite rise as high as we were before the first dip. With each subsequent health challenge that takes us down, our recovery is less complete.

Physicians are familiar with the pattern. You may have seen it in your own aging parents. The thought of taking this thrill ride yourself can be depressing.

Is this an "accept the aging I cannot change" thing? Not necessarily.

Although in his seventies, a neighbor of mine was a picture of health—outgoing, energetic, and enjoying life. He played golf, tennis, table tennis, bocce, and pool. He was known for his broad smiles, quick wit, and good humor.

Two years ago, he suffered a life-threatening infection in his heart. Suddenly, he found himself hospitalized with his survival not assured. In a last ditch effort, doctors performed open-heart surgery. They managed to save his life.

When I saw him weeks later, he seemed a shadow of his former self. It reminded me of the changes I saw in my father after his quadruple bypass.

As my dad recovered from his heart attack and surgery, he was weak and unsure of himself. He seemed mentally slower. He struggled with anxiety and was briefly addicted to tranquilizers. After knowing my father as an independent and self-confident man, this was painful to watch.

With both my neighbor and my father, my first impression was that they had begun a serious downward spiral from which they would never recover. In both cases, I was wrong.

Following his surgery, I moved in with my father and encouraged him to fight back. Walks around the living room became walks around the block—and then walks around the lake. He kicked his medication habit through sheer force of will.

Dad then became a "meals on wheels" volunteer, providing nourishment and a friendly face to needy seniors. He even became a relief caregiver for a neighbor woman whose husband was in the final stages of Alzheimer's disease. In many ways, my father was healthier than before his heart attack.

I have seen similar changes in my neighbor. In the last twenty-four hours, I happened to play both bocce ball and table tennis with him. He beat me in both. His energy, infectious smile, and sense of humor have returned. It is great to see the strength of his recovery.

Rollercoaster rides may catch us by surprise—but they don't have to be the last ride we take.

Odds and Ends

Following are some brief comments about a few other health concerns that are common in aging adults.

Shingles is an infection that is most likely to occur between the ages of fifty and seventy. The same virus that causes chickenpox is responsible. In fact, after a person recovers from chickenpox, the virus may lay dormant in nerves near the spinal cord for decades.

Later, when the immune system is compromised by illness, drugs, inadequate nutrition, stress, or even aging itself, the virus becomes active. It then travels down nerves to the skin where it can cause a painful, blistering rash.

The rash usually appears on only one side of the body and is preceded by abnormal sensations such as pain, burning, "pins and needles," itching, numbness, or sensitivity to touch. After the rash breaks out, the virus may continue to spread and occasionally cause serious problems, including paralysis or vision loss.

About one in three people will develop shingles in their lifetime. The shingles vaccine is known to cut the risk of the disease in half and lessen symptoms in those who still become affected.

If diagnosed within three days of the rash's appearance, antiviral drugs can aid recovery. Corticosteroids and other drugs may help with symptom relief.

Osteoporosis means "porous bones." This level of bone density loss eventually affects only 3% of Americans—eighty percent of them women. Larger percentages have *osteopenia*, low bone density that may become osteoporosis. Loss of bone density means bones are more likely to break. Each year, over two million U. S. elderly break bones—usually due to falls.

Bone density increases until about age thirty. After this, the process is reversed as more bone is broken down than replaced. Hormones play a role, with menopause triggering a rapid decline in bone density in many women. Once considered an unavoidable part of aging, we now know that osteoporosis is both preventable and treatable.

To keep bones healthy requires a supply of minerals (mainly calcium and phosphorus) and vitamin D. Given adequate nutrition, the most effective preventative step is to engage in regular weight-bearing exercises such as walking, stair climbing, dancing, or weight training.

For those diagnosed with osteoporosis, hormone replacement therapy may be considered. Prescription medications are also available to help reverse bone loss.

Teeth and Gums are not immune to the effects of aging. A decline in motivation and dexterity often reduce brushing and flossing as we age, to the detriment of our oral hygiene. Only about 25% of us will manage to keep a majority of our natural teeth after age seventy-five.

Teeth become more vulnerable as they accumulate cracks and other damage. Grinding and clenching of teeth during deep sleep can accelerate tooth loss. Using a mouth guard at night can reduce the abrasive damage.

Teeth can also be lost because of underlying bone loss. Surprisingly, however, the greatest risk of tooth loss comes not from tooth damage or bone loss, but from gum disease. Gums naturally recede with age, increasing the chances of plaque formation, inflammation, and low-grade infection. Along with brushing and flossing, regular cleanings by a hygienist help fight this *periodontal disease.*

Diet plays a significant role in healthy aging. This is because our digestive system is not as forgiving as it once was. For example, if a young person gets inadequate amounts of calcium in their diet, the body copes by increasing calcium absorption. The body of an older person loses this adaptive ability. We even lose some of our normal absorptive capacity. Balanced nutrition becomes essential.

Increasing fiber and water intake (along with exercise) can reduce the incidence of constipation—a frequent complaint of the elderly.

Overeating is one of the main causes of health problems in older adults. A slowed metabolism is not so forgiving of excess calorie intake. Overeating may be partly due to a decrease in taste and smell sensitivities.

A *body mass index* of less than 25 is the goal. (BMI calculators can be found online.)

Thyroid Disorders are not a normal part of aging. Recognizing symptoms, however, can lead to effective treatments when the thyroid is not functioning properly.

The thyroid is a bilobed gland that sits in the neck just in front of the windpipe. Its primary job is to produce hormones that regulate *metabolism*—the speed of vital body functions.

In *hypothyroidism*, the thyroid gland does not produce adequate amounts of hormone. Fewer than 5% of older people have this condition. Women are affected twice as often as men. Sometimes when the body attempts to respond to the inadequacy of thyroid hormone, the thyroid gland will enlarge—a condition called *goiter*.

A lack of thyroid hormone can cause a laundry list of symptoms including confusion, decreased appetite, weight loss, cold sensitivity, constipation, joint stiffness, dizziness, fatigue, and weakness. The skin may become dry and coarse, the face puffy and swollen—especially around the eyes.

Treatment involves taking replacement thyroid hormone. It may take several months of gradually increasing doses to determine the correct prescription. Such replacement is usually very effective, but must be continued for life.

Hyperthyroidism is the overproduction of thyroid hormone, which can speed up body functions. Only 2% of older adults have this condition. Hyperthyroidism is sometimes a result of Graves' disease—when antibodies stimulate thyroid activity. In other cases, small nodules grow on the thyroid gland, increasing the production of thyroid hormone.

The most common symptoms of hyperthyroidism are weight loss and fatigue. A variety of other symptoms may accompany the condition, including abnormal heart rhythms, anxiety, and trembling of the hands.

Treatments may involve surgery to remove a portion of the thyroid, or radioactive iodine that kills thyroid gland cells. Replacement thyroid hormone may be required to achieve a proper balance after these interventions. In almost all cases, hyperthyroidism can be cured and symptoms eliminated.

Low Back Pain is one of the most common complaints that bring people to the doctor's office. About 80% of people are affected at some point in their lives. It is most often the result of muscle and joint strains that usually respond well to rest and mild pain medications. Up to 90% of patients report being completely better within six weeks.

Because of this, imaging (with X-rays, CT scans, or MRI's) is not recommended after an initial consultation for common back pain. Fewer than 1% of such tests identify the cause of the problem. Only when pain becomes chronic (12 weeks) or other health "red flags" are present would a search for underlying anatomical problems be advised. Musculoskeletal issues including osteoarthritis, herniated disk, compressed nerves, or fractures may sometimes produce lower back pain.

Obesity, lack of exercise, stress, poor posture, and poor sleeping conditions are common causes of low back pain. Weight loss, regular walking, core strengthening, computer or chair adjustment, and mattress replacement are often effective preventative measures. My son-in-law, whose job involves heavy lifting, swears by Yoga for back pain relief.

Physical changes in the back with aging include loss of flexibility in muscles and discs, loss of muscle strength, and decreased ability to absorb the significant physical forces that affect the back. The risk of injury thus increases.

Bed rest may actually make pain worse. Resuming normal activities as soon as possible usually leads to quicker recovery. Stretching and strengthening exercises should begin when they do not aggravate pain.

Women may experience low back pain in response to serious medical conditions of the reproductive system including endometriosis, ovarian cysts, uterine fibroids, and cancer. In both men and women, low back pain may be symptomatic of serious health issues. It should not be ignored if it becomes chronic or severe.

In most cases, low back pain will subside. This is the time to begin focusing on prevention of recurrence through conditioning and improved habits.

Music and Laughter

After all this discussion of disease and deterioration, here are two pleasant suggestions:

Listen to music every day.
Laugh every day.

Along with exercise and sensible diet, there may not be a better prescription for healthy living.

Research indicates that **music** may:

-- *Ease pain* by stimulating the release of dopamine and endorphins. (For example, patients recovering from surgery require less pain medication if they are listening to music.)

-- *Improve blood vessel function*, which increases blood flow.

-- *Aid recovery from brain damage* because rhythms and melodies stimulate familiar neurological patterns.

-- *Stimulate immune function*, helping to fight disease.

-- *Promote production of biochemical stress-relievers,* which may aid sleep, reduces anxiety, combats depression, lift mood, and improve cognitive performance.

Laughter has similar positive effects. It has been shown to *lower blood pressure, improve cardiac health, and reduce stress hormones.* It also *activates T-cells (white blood cells) to enhance immunity.* Of course, the positive effects of laughter on mood is obvious. If not the *best* medicine, it is certainly a *good* medicine.

****

You can live to be a hundred if you give up all things that make you want to live to be a hundred.

Woody Allen

People ask me what I'd most appreciate getting for my eighty-seventh birthday. I tell them, a paternity suit.

George Burns

I don't plan to grow old gracefully. I plan to have face-lifts until my ears meet.

Rita Rudner

While I had often said that I wanted to die in bed, what I really meant was that in my old age I wanted to be stepped on by an elephant while making love.

Roger Zelazny

An archeologist is the best husband a woman can have.
The older she gets, the more interested he is in her.

Agatha Christie

I'm at the age when my back goes out more than I do.

Phyllis Diller

We could certainly slow the aging process down if it had to work its way through Congress.

Will Rogers

Grandpa is driving down the freeway to visit his young grandchildren when the car phone rings. Answering, he hears his daughter's voice urgently warning him.

"Dad, I just heard on the news that there is a car going the wrong way on Interstate 80. Please be careful."

"Heck," Grandpa replies, "It's not just one car—it's hundreds of them!"

Resilience

In concluding *Section I: Body Blows*, I want to emphasize the word *resilience*. Reading about all the challenges and diseases in the elderly can be disheartening. But, I am a "glass half full" kind of person. **Nearly every health issue of old age can be prevented, postponed, or healed.**

The tissues and organs of our body have a remarkable capacity for regeneration and restoration, even in our later years. Keep in mind that most cells in our body are replaced regularly, many in a matter of days to months. We are always rejuvenating. Often our healing just requires some extra rest, modification of daily habits, and time.

I have had many health issues that have demonstrated my body's resilience. I have talked about several of them in these essays. Another example was a debilitating case of *plantar fasciitis*—a very painful inflammation of the bottom of the heel. At its worst, I experienced shooting pain as I walked on it, especially first thing in the morning. I had to give up jogging. I could not walk barefoot. I thought I would never play sports again.

This condition lasted for months, and I accepted it as an ongoing part of my life. Then one day I realized that it was gone.

I have been careful to wear supportive shoes and keep my exercise low impact. As a result, I have not had any issue with plantar fasciitis for many years. What a summer pleasure to kick off my shoes and go barefoot!

Similarly, I have had knees that would swell with exertion, tendinitis in my elbows, a weak and painful thumb joint, etc. The conditions stemmed from the injuries of overuse and lack of proper conditioning. In each case, I thought the damage was permanent, only to realize after months (even years) that it had healed.

Just last week, I helped lift a 135 pound BBQ grill out of a truck. That night, pain began radiating from my shoulder to the point that I could not sleep. The pain was debilitating for several days. Visions of rotator cuff surgery danced in my head. After a week of rest, ice treatments, and ibuprofen, my shoulder is working pain-free.

Perhaps the most surprising example of healing I have experienced involved swollen tendons in the palm of my hand. My doctor diagnosed it as Dupuytren's Contracture, a disease that gradually pulls the fingers forward to the point that they cannot be straightened. Progression often leads to surgery.

Now three years later, the swelling is almost entirely gone. There is a strong hereditary component of Dupuytren's. Certainly, it could begin progressing again at any time. Still, I am amazed and grateful that my body is not giving up without a fight.

I end this essay with a final reminder:

If it doesn't look right, feel right or work right, get it checked!

Then, whatever the diagnosis, *trust in the powerful synergy of modern medicine and your body's natural resilience.*

Epilogue 1

"To me, old age is always 15 years older than I am."

                                        - Francis Bacon

There have been two meta-themes in Section I:

1. Aging is natural, unavoidable, and not always pleasant.
2. Our habits, choices, and attitude can prevent or slow many aspects of aging.

With regard to theme 1.

There is some chance that the word *unavoidable* will have to be replaced in future editions of this book. Scientists are making remarkable progress in understanding the fundamental causes of aging. This produces the tantalizing possibility that aging may someday be considered a treatable condition, one that at least can be significantly delayed.

Unfortunately, future breakthroughs in longevity research may produce another distinction for Baby Boomers. We may be the last generation without access to drugs and procedures that can artificially extend life. Bummer.

We should, however, always count our blessings. At least we weren't eaten by a lion. At least we didn't die of smallpox, polio, or plague. At least we will have self-driving cars when we lose our coordination and eyesight. Looking back on human history, we have much for which to be grateful.

The fact that the longevity revolution will probably come too late for us only intensifies the urgency for us to take care of ourselves.

This brings me to theme 2.

Most of the suggestions I have offered in Section 1 are not new information to you. We are perhaps the first fully health conscious generation. So why are so many of us overweight and underexercised? Why is it often so difficult to do the things that will give us the best chance of remaining healthy? Blame biological evolution and corporate evolution.

We are biologically programmed (think genes) to crave sugar, fat, and salt. Our ancient ancestors had to find those resources to stay alive. Now our bodies crave them in an environment where they are easily accessible.

Corporations understand our cravings and have evolved to satisfy them. Foods are invented, modified, and advertised with one goal in mind—increased sales and profits. This is "product natural selection."

Conserving energy is also a survival adaptation—and modern life allows most of us to be sedentary. Clearly, the odds are stacked against us.

I am no health saint. I work to overcome my inertia in doing the things I should (like exercising). I work to control my desires to indulge in things I shouldn't (like potato chips and milk chocolate). To aid my willpower while keeping life fun, I choose the philosophy "all good things in moderation."

If you struggle with the maintenance of good health habits as I do, the following may be helpful:

-- *Make it fun.* It is difficult to stick with any diet or exercise program if you don't enjoy it. (The best exercise is the one you will do!) Try new sports. Exercise to music.

-- *Get into a routine.* Positive habits can be as addicting as bad habits.

-- *Start slowly.* Nothing defeats an exercise resolution faster than an injury. Also, be realistic about your weight loss goals. One or two pounds a month is healthy.

-- *Don't give up.* You will have lapses. Just start again.

-- *Keep a record.* This can add motivation.

-- *Celebrate incremental achievements.* Challenge yourself to small goals, and then reward yourself.

-- *Work with a spouse, partner, or friend.* Some will find this very motivating and supportive. (Introverts like me may put on headphones and enjoy "alone time" at the gym.)

-- *Spend the money for professional help.* Think how much illness or injury can cost. Invest in yourself.

I wish you good luck and good health.

****

Longevity Research

Scientists have discovered that certain gene variations are more common in long-lived humans. One such gene has been designated *daf-2*. It produces proteins that help cells respond to IGF-1, a growth hormone. By artificially mutating the daf-2 gene, researchers have been able to double the healthy lifespan in *C-elegans* worms and extend the lives of mice as well.

Our body cells respond to dozens of hormone-like messaging molecules in the blood (like the one produced by the daf-2 gene). Messaging molecule concentrations change as the body ages.

The blood of young individuals—whether mice or humans—contains messaging molecules that *keep cells youthful and healthy*. The blood of older individuals contains different messaging molecules that cause cells to age and eventually die. This has profound implications.

It would seem logical that if we can just bathe our cells in the right chemical cocktail of messaging molecules, we may keep them functioning at a youthful level. In what are destined to become classic experiments, old mice were given a continuous supply of young mouse blood. Aging in the old mice *was reversed*—as measured in tissues of the muscle, pancreas, liver, heart, and brain.

Messaging molecules are very consistent across species. When old mice are continuously given young *human* blood, it also reverses the aging process.

There is some preliminary evidence that intermittent fasting or calorie restriction may affect the messaging molecules of aging in a positive direction. (It is too early to recommend drastic lifestyle changes based on this research.)

Scientists are currently isolating and identifying these messaging factors. There is every reason to believe that when the genetics and biochemistry of aging is fully understood, we will find ways to extend human life—perhaps substantially.

One day, the question may not be *how long will I live*, but rather *how long do I **want** to live.*

(Please Note: As of this writing, I am not aware of *any* commercially available product or procedure that represents the Fountain of Youth for humans. Anti-aging promises will certainly be made by corporations long before they are clinically supported. Stay smart and skeptical.)

Maximizing Our Heredity

Question: Since most of the health challenges of aging have a genetic component, why bother improving our health habits?

Answer: Statistics.

It is true that marathon runners have heart attacks and non-smokers get lung cancer. However, statistics show that people who exercise regularly have significantly *decreased chances* of heart disease and non-smokers have dramatically *decreased chances* of developing lung cancer. Positive health habits are all about moving the *odds* of healthy aging in our favor.

116

Part of the positive effect of health habits stems from a surprising fact: *Our health habits and mental attitude influence our genes.*

About 23,000 genes control each human cell. This is our unalterable heredity. But these genes represent only 4% of the DNA coiled into our chromosomes. Other portions of our DNA are involved in gene *regulation*—the promoting or inhibiting of gene expression. This regulatory DNA (that turns genes on and off) is influenced by the chemical environment of each cell (the hormones and other messaging molecules that flow through our body). For example, two people may have inherited the same disease-causing gene, but the gene may only be expressed in the person with a stress hormone circulating in their blood.

The study of how environmental factors regulate our genes is a relatively young field of science called *epigenetics.* Its discoveries are beginning to answer the question "How do lifestyle choices increase our chances for good health?" What has been observed is constant communication between the environment of the cell and the DNA within the cell. Our diet, exercise patterns, stress levels, *expectations*, and other factors (which we control) actually influence which genes are expressed and which genes are turned off.

We have all heard that keeping a positive attitude promotes health and helps us fight disease. Now scientists are understanding the biochemistry that moves this notion from wishful thinking to biological reality. Whether it originates from religious faith, pop psychology, or personal philosophy, positive thinking is translated into physiological changes in the body. *Our mental attitude can affect the type and levels of messaging molecules in our blood, which in turn affects gene expression and how cells function.*

Let me share a startling example from the scientific literature. Dr. Becca Levy is Professor of Epidemiology at Yale University. Her research evaluated data from the *Ohio Longitudinal Study of Aging,* which followed 660 people for 23 years. She and her colleagues found that *those who had positive expectations about growing older lived an average of 7.5 years longer than those who held negative stereotypes about aging.* **In fact, the perception of aging influenced longevity more than blood pressure, cholesterol, body mass index, or the tendency to exercise.**

117

The *Baltimore Longitudinal Study of Aging* similarly demonstrated that *people who maintained a positive attitude about aging improved their memory by 30% and reduced their risk of a cardiovascular event by 80%.*

This understanding of how the cell environment affects cell DNA has been a revelation. Let me summarize:

We can influence the activity of our genes by our lifestyle choices and mental attitude.

Because of this, at least some of our genetic susceptibility to aging and disease is modifiable.

All that we think, feel, and experience at every moment influences our gene activity—affecting our health, wellbeing, and lifespan.

(These hope-inspiring findings are detailed in a book called *Super Genes: Unlock the Astonishing Power of Your DNA for Optimum Health and Well-Being*. In this 2015 publication, Deepak Chopra, M.D. and Rudolph Tanzi, Ph.D. discuss the epigenetic findings that can promote our well-being and extend our "healthspan.")

The oldest of our generation have recently turned seventy. (Remember when sixty-four seemed ancient? The Beatles wondered if we would be needed—or even fed—at such an age!)

It is true, we have more yesterdays than tomorrows.

But consider the following:

Cornelius Vanderbilt began buying railroads at age 70.

Katsusuke Yanagisawa climbed Mt. Everest at age 71.

Oscar Swahn earned an Olympic silver medal at age 72.

Peter Roget invented the thesaurus at age 73.

Ferdinand de Lesseps was building the Suez Canal at age 74.

Nelson Mandela was elected S. African President at age 75.

Grandma Moses started painting at age 76.

John Glenn became the oldest person in space at age 77.

Justice O. Wendell Holmes clarified the first amendment at 78.

John Powanda became oldest Peace Corps volunteer at 79.

Sir George Martin produced the Beatles album *Love* at 80.

Ben Franklin insured the passage of the Constitution at 81.

Churchill wrote *History of English Speaking People* at 82.

Dr. Benjamin Spock was arrested at a peace protest at 83.

W. Somerset Maugham wrote *Points of View* at 84.

Coco Chanel was still running her fashion company at 85.

Katherine Pelton set age group record in 200-m. butterfly at 86.

Mary Baker Eddy founded The Christian Science Monitor at 87.

Michelangelo drafted plans for Santa Maria Church at 88.

Arthur Rubinstein performed in Carnegie Hall at 89.

Chagall became first living artist to be exhibited at Louvre at 90.

Adolph Zukon was chairman of Paramount Pictures at 91.

Paul Spangler completed his fourteenth marathon at 92.

Strom Thurmond won reelection to the US Senate at 93.

George Burns performed standup comedy in N.Y. at 94.

Martha Graham was still choreographing dance at 95.

Harry Bernstein published *The Invisible Wall* at 96.

Bertrand Russell continued to write extensively at 97.

Beatrice Wood continued to create ceramics at 98.

Teiichi Igarashi climbed Mt. Fuji at 99.

Grandma Moses continued to paint masterpieces at 100.

And don't forget George H.W. Bush skydiving on his 90th birthday! So does this make the rest of us underachievers? Of course not. These are exceptional people doing exceptional things at exceptional ages. The point is, age alone does not have to *limit* us.

Beliefs about aging may be more powerful than our genes in determining our *experience* of aging. For this reason, we owe it to ourselves to redefine our expectations.

Let's forget our memories of how previous generations have aged. (They were living up to their own expectations.)

Let's throw out our stereotypes of what it means to grow old. (We need not set limits to our own potential.)

We can be *exceptional* in ways that do not make the record books. We can be *extraordinary* in our ability to live with purpose:

-- caring for our spouse and loved ones
-- loving our children and grandchildren
-- serving our friends and community
-- sharing our creativity
-- continuing to learn, grow, and achieve

By maximizing our health, we Boomers can continue to change the world—while reinventing what it means to age.

———————

I'm keyed to keep groovin'.
                                   Far out, man!

Can you dig it?
                                   You're blowin' my mnd.

What a trip!
                                   The grooviest.

I'm TCB.
                                   Outtasight!

Right on.

(Did any of us ever really talk like this?)

Section II

Memories and Musings

These are my memories and musings.
They may stimulate some of yours.
Reflection is encouraged.
Nostalgia is optional.

The stories you are about to read are true. (as memory allows)
Some names have been changed to protect the innocent. (me!)

A Journey to Remember

It was Sunday morning October 4, 1959. I was twelve years old. I remember being very nervous—but determined. I just had to do it.

I did not ask Mom or Dad for permission. Mom would have thought it was too dangerous. Dad would have just thought I was nuts. I don't think I could have explained it to them. The motivation came from a place in me that I could not describe in words.

Here is the back-story:

I lived the first six years of my life in Bell Gardens, California. In the middle of first grade, we moved to Whittier where I would grow into adulthood. For a long time after the move, I would *intentionally* remember the people and events of my first neighborhood before drifting off to sleep each night. I didn't want the memories to fade.

First, I usually remembered my friend Joe. After our morning kindergarten class let out, he and I would walk down to the high school where the students were out front during their lunch break. In my nightly reverie, I could see the teenagers sitting in circles on the lawn and clustered on the front steps of the auditorium. In my mind, I could hear the music that blared from the loudspeakers, songs like "You Belong to Me" by Jo Stafford and "Cry" by Johnnie Ray. I also could visualize the old beat-up food truck that parked right across the street from the school.

Joe and I would bounce from group to group, collecting soda pop bottles from the students until our little arms were full. Then we would run them across the street to the lunch wagon where the man would give us a penny for each bottle we returned.

One day as Joe leapt off the curb with another load of treasure, he was hit by a car. I remember the students screaming. Eventually, an ambulance arrived and I heard someone say that the little boy was dead.

When the police arrived, they asked me if I knew where Joe lived. I took them to the house and stood outside while the police told Joe's mom that her son had been killed. I do not remember crying. I remember feeling sad that my friend was gone, but my strongest reactions were of confusion and uncertainty. I knew it was a major event to have your friend die, but I did not know what I was supposed to do.

My parents did not know what to say. We did not attend the funeral and Joe was not mentioned around our house anymore.

In my bedtime review, it was important to remember Joe.

I also remembered my friend Danny. We built a raft out of scrap wood. We used it to cross the "pond" that appeared by the railroad tracks after a winter storm. Danny was a year or two older and the leader of our "club."

One day Danny had the idea that each of us should pass a test to be official members. He led us to the high school football stadium. He explained that if we wanted to stay in the group we must demonstrate our courage and commitment—by sliding down the steel girder that supported the stands.

We scrambled up the stairs to look over the back railing of the stadium. I was terrified. I thought that I would certainly fall and die with a splat on the asphalt below.

Danny went first, fearless as usual. He slid down quickly and hopped off the beam at the bottom just to emphasize how easy it was. With Danny yelling encouragement from below, the others followed one after the other until I was the last left on top. I was petrified with fear, but being in the "club" seemed vital. I forced myself—with tears streaming down my face—over the rail. I inched down with eyes closed, gripping the beam with all of my trembling six-year-old strength.

In my memory time, I could re-experience both the terror and the triumph of this "rite of passage."

So the journey upon which I was about to embark was all about the memories. I had to return to their source. I was determined to visit my early childhood home.

Mom would occasionally drive us to doctor appointments in our old neighborhood, so I memorized the route. I knew it was a long way, but it was not until years later that I measured the distance in my car—over 25 miles round trip. Mom and Dad would have been right. It was dangerous and I was probably nuts.

My vehicle was an old balloon tire bicycle that had been a Christmas gift several years before. The red and silver paint was chipped, the multicolored plastic streamers attached to the handlebar grips were badly faded. The horn—that had been such an important accessory when the bike was new—no longer worked.

I had to mow the lawn first so that Dad would not start wondering where I was. Once my chores were done, it was not unusual for me to leave the house and spend the day playing with friends. I don't remember if I told my Mom a lie or if I just took off without saying anything. It was late morning when I pulled the back door shut, climbed on my bike, and started riding.

I had saved a little money from my allowance so that when I reached my old street corner I could get some fries and a strawberry shake at the old burger place. My heart was racing with excitement.

Much of the ride was along major highways where the drivers were not used to looking out for bikes. Long sections of road had no curbs or sidewalks. I felt relief each time I made it to the next gas station where I could get off the street for a minute and get a drink of cold water from the fountain.

After two o'clock, it seemed like all of the gas stations had the World Series on TV, so I followed the progress of the game as I rode. It was the first World Series game ever played in Los Angeles as the Dodgers hosted the Chicago White Sox. Don Drysdale was pitching for LA and the whole town was watching or listening.

The familiar voice of Vin Scully was somehow comforting, but I became quite nervous as I left the residential neighborhoods and passed through dirty oil fields and industrial areas. I felt like I was on the road to Oz with unknown dangers lurking around every corner. My anxiety grew in direct proportion to my distance from home, but I had dreamed of this journey for too many nights to turn back now.

126

I finally began to see some familiar landmarks that told me I was nearing my destination. I stood up on my bike and pedaled faster. Soon I could see my old street with the same burger joint on the corner. I had done it.

My joy soon faded as I turned down the street and realized that things looked unfamiliar. I wasn't even sure which house had been ours. The neighborhood that had always brought warmth and comfort in my nightly review now felt cold and threatening.

What was I thinking? Nothing was as I remembered. I rode down to the train tracks. The "pond" that we had sailed was nothing more than a filthy little ditch next to the rails. I rode over to the high school. The stadium that seemed so imposing was just a standard set of bleachers. Everything was still there, but nothing matched my memories.

I wondered if I could find Danny. I thought about how great it would be to see him again. Would he know me? Would he remember me the way I remembered him? Now I was feeling very nervous again.

I picked out a house that I thought was his. Before I could make my move, the front door opened and fear shot down my spine. A young woman with a baby in her arms was bending down to pick something up off the front porch. Was this Danny's mom? Danny's sister? I realized I didn't even know his last name. I wasn't sure what to do or what to say. She looked up and noticed me. I was frozen.

"Does Danny live here?" I finally blurted out.

The woman seemed puzzled. After hesitating, she responded, "No Danny here."

"Thanks" I managed. I quickly rode off— deflated.

It was mid-afternoon and I realized I was hungry. Time for fries and a strawberry shake I thought. My mouth began to water, but then I wondered—would this just be another disappointment?

I ordered at the burger place on the corner. The fries were crisp, golden brown, and thick enough so that the middle of each fry stayed steamy hot for a long time. The shake was creamy with the strong aroma of strawberries. I could feel the texture of strawberry pieces and little seeds on my tongue. I would eat a hot fry with salt and ketchup and quickly put out the fire in my mouth with a spoonful of thick, cold shake.

It was *just* as I remembered. There was some consolation to be found in hot fries and a cold shake.

The journey home seemed much quicker. The closer I got, the faster I pedaled and the better I felt. I made it home in time for dinner. No questions were asked.

Don Drysdale had succeeded in defeating Chicago 3-1 to give the Dodgers the Series lead on their way to the championship. I had succeeded in overcoming my fears and following through on my long-standing desire to visit my memories. I did not think much about Bell Gardens after this. It did not seem important anymore.

-- Which of your childhood memories stand out?
-- When was the last time you dug out the old photos and spent some time reflecting?
-- Have you shared your memories with your kids & grandkids? (The memory prompts at the end of this book may help.)

Mom and Dad

I picked the right parents. I did not realize this until I was older and heard others talk about their childhoods. In our household, there was no physical abuse, no verbal abuse, no neglect, and no drunkenness. My parents were just straight-forward, genuine, caring, responsible, and supportive. I would say they were normal, but I am beginning to wonder if they were not exceptional instead.

Dad worked regular hours as a draftsman, engineering and drawing piping plans for hospitals and oil refineries. On weekends, he did projects around the house and yard. Because he had worked hard as a child on the family farm, he expected my brother and me to participate in household chores and take on responsibilities as we grew. He was clearly the authority figure in our household. He could be demanding at times, but he was a patient teacher and treated us fairly.

Mom had been a secretary before she married, but took on the (then) typical role of homemaker after I was born. She was always there for us as mother, chef, nurse, and chauffeur. She took an interest in my schoolwork—helping me improve my atrocious penmanship in elementary school and proof-reading my papers in high school.

I think back on our family life with great warmth and gratitude. What a fortunate way to grow up.

As I experienced parenthood myself, my appreciation for my own parents grew. One year I wrote a thank you note to my Dad in honor of Father's Day. I did not realize how much it would mean to him. He had my words framed. They hung prominently in his living room until the day he died.

Thank You Dad

Dear Dad,

Thank you for working so hard fifty weeks a year, year after year. You gave me the chance to grow up in a nice neighborhood where I felt safe and secure. You made it possible for Mom to be there every day when I came home from school, to drive me to swim lessons or the library, and to have the time to be our Cub Scout den mother. I was able to attend good schools and have the positive experiences that come from after school sports and Boy Scout campouts. Thanks for being such a good provider for our family.

Thank you for spending your precious one or two-week vacations taking us on family trips that always seemed to turn into family adventures. Who could forget being caught on the wrong side of the lake in a lightning storm or coming grill-to grill with a huge logging truck on a narrow mountain road? You taught me that exploring can be both scary and fun —and that the best memories are unplanned.

Thank you for teaching me how to do things, like changing a bike tire or checking the oil in the car. Thanks to you, I know how to use a square to line up boards at right angles and how to pound in nails without bending them. Of course, you also showed me how to cover any construction mistakes with trim strip! You taught me the secrets of making Morgan pancakes and Morgan cookies. And thanks for teaching me to be skeptical about the things I read or hear. Your cautious and questioning attitude will always be with me when I listen to a politician or see an ad on TV.

Thank you for teaching me all the things you didn't know you were teaching—like how to laugh at life. There was a lot of laughter in our house, and not just from the bad jokes that you brought home from work. You found the humor in everyday situations and you taught us how to laugh at ourselves. I remember the time we drove all the way to the mountains to have a wiener roast, only to discover when we got there that you and Mom each thought the other had packed the hot dogs! We still laughed and had a good time eating empty buns with our chips and cooking marshmallows for dessert. It seemed that no matter the situation, we could always laugh at ourselves and see the humor in life's frustrations.

Thank you for teaching me the real meaning of caring and commitment. I will always remember how you cared for Mom every day for months, then years as she struggled with her illnesses. You bore the burden as the caregiver for such a long time and I never heard you complain. Your personal strength and dedication will always be an inspiration to me. You taught me that the real meaning of love shows through when the times are the most difficult.

Thank you for living your life with integrity and teaching me the meaning of the word by your example. You spoke the truth without trying to use words to manipulate. You treated others with fairness and expected them to do the same. I never saw you try to take advantage of anyone. You have a strong sense of what is right and what is wrong and have always been willing to stand up for the right. By any standard that I can think of, you are a good man. I have always respected you for the simple virtues that today seem so rare.

I hope these few words will let you know that all your efforts have not gone unnoticed or unappreciated. Thanks for all you are and all you have taught me. Thanks for being the kind of man that a son can be proud to call his father.

I love you.

Your Grateful Son

Unfortunately, I never wrote a similar note for my Mom while she was alive. If I could write to her today, I would want to say:

Thank You Mom

Dear Mom,

Thanks for taking me to swimming lessons. Thanks for taking me to piano lessons. Thanks for changing my wet sheets every night without making me feel like a failure. Thanks for rubbing Vicks on my chest. Thanks for sending me to sixth-grade camp. Thanks for fixing me a brown bag lunch for school every day with pb&j, baloney, or tuna sandwiches. Thanks for letting me leave my Lionel Train and Lincoln Logs all over the living room floor. Thanks for being Cub Scout Den Mother. Thanks for not killing me after I teased my brother mercilessly for hours. Thanks for giving me the freedom to explore. Thanks for telling me that eighth-grade dance class would be fun. Thanks for teaching me how to tie a tie. Thanks for picking me up every night after basketball practice. Thanks for coming to all of my high school games. Thanks for buying me my varsity jacket and sewing on the letter. Thanks for letting me drive your car to school when you did not need it. Thanks for all of the great dinners for which I never said thanks. Thanks for introducing me to all kinds of music. Thanks for telling me I was smart. Thanks for not yelling when I used all of the hot water for my shower.

Thanks for sending me hometown newspaper clippings and boxes of homemade cookies when I was a freshman at Stanford. Thanks for not laughing (too hard) when all of my underwear turned pink in the wash with my new red Stanford sweatshirt. Thanks for...everything.

What a gift you have given me. Not just the gift of life— the gift of feeling your unconditional love through all of these years. I am so grateful.

I live with few regrets, but I do regret we did not have more time together. Perhaps I just did not take advantage of the time we had.
I want to know about your childhood, your dreams, and your disappointments.
I want to know about your thoughts and feelings, your insights and wisdom.
I never asked you the important questions and now I will never know your answers.
I do know your heart, your gentle ways, and your nurturing kindness.

For all you have given me, I am so thankful.

I will always love you.

-- Parents are not perfect. Focus on their positive qualities when you think of them. Express appreciation if you still can.
-- What are your best memories of your parents?

Were You Raised In a Barn?

Both of my parents grew up on farms. I loved their language. They said things like:

Your room is a pigsty.
Hold your horses.
He couldn't hit the broad side of a barn.
Let's make hay while the sun shines.
Don't look a gift horse in the mouth.
That'll be a tough row to hoe.
Stop runnin' around like a chicken with its head cut off.
Don't change horses in the middle of the stream.
You look happy as a pig in slop.
That's like finding a needle in a haystack.
I'm cold as a frog's behind.
Don't beat a dead horse.
He's dumb as a fence post.
I was naked as a jaybird.
We're livin' high on the hog.
You look like something the cat dragged in.
Put on your Sunday-go-t'-meetin' clothes.
I was so broke, I didn't have two nickels to rub together.
She was madder than a wet hen.
Don't put the cart before the horse.
An empty wagon makes the most noise.
Were you raised in a barn?

-- Did your parents have regional or ethnic language favorites?

135

My Second Mom

My former mother-in-law has been a second mom to me. She is 92 and going strong. I asked her if she had any advice about aging. She shared the following:

Expect surprises. Nothing stays the same. Your reaction to aging will probably be: ARE YOU KIDDING ME!?

Find a good doctor, one that you have confidence in and can relate to. Keep shopping until you find one that will take time for you and truly hear you.

Volunteer to do something that interests you.

Make friends from various backgrounds. Learn to listen without judging. Be interested in them and open about yourself.

Take care of old hurts and disappointments. It may take a lot of talking and crying, but you need to release the tension. Anger is bad—it causes the body to tighten-up. Find a way to let it go.

Love and accept yourself. Continue to learn about yourself. It has taken me a long time to believe that I am O.K.

A close friend of mine died. I used to cry every time I drove past her house. Then one day, I didn't cry. Time allowed me to work through it without knowing how.

Realize we are not fully in charge. If you find a spiritual connection you are fortunate—it either happens or it doesn't—but it can bring you peace.

The most important advice I can give about aging is to adjust your attitude. Focus on gratitude. It's like I am watching my own movie. There are sad parts when I have to cry, but there are many more scenes that are heartwarming. I have lived such a blessed life.

Adventures in Childhood

My parents were raised in wide open spaces, Dad in Kansas and Mom in Nebraska. As they began to raise their family, they wanted to live as far from the LA city center as Dad's daily commute would allow. East Whittier was the edge of suburbia when we moved into our new three-bedroom tract house in 1953.

The area had a friendly small town feeling. I remember the milkman stopping his truck to give my brother and me free bottles of cold chocolate milk. He tried to convince us that he had milked a brown cow to secure our treat. The owner of the Frosty Freeze gave us free "baby cones" when we animatedly faked starvation. The mechanic at the gas station sometimes opened the coke machine to hand us a free bottle on a hot day. It was the land of Ozzie and Harriet.

Our neighborhood was surrounded by orange groves and open fields that begged to be explored. Near our house was a road that went over some rolling hills. My friends and I would challenge each other to see who could ride their bikes down the steep inclines without "chickening out" by putting on our brakes. I can still remember the wind on my face and the scary vibrations of the bike as it picked up speed.

Sometimes we enhanced the experience by using clothespins to attach playing cards to our bike frame. The cards clicked on the spokes—and in my childhood imagination, I was riding atop a powerful motorcycle.

Imagination also had a downside. In order to get to the steep hills, we had to ride past the perilous "bamboo forest." This was a swampy area beside the railroad tracks, which—

according to the older boys—was the home of bloodthirsty hobos. We peddled as fast as we could with fear in our throats to avoid being grabbed off our bikes by the unseen killers.

Mom and Dad gave me a good deal of freedom. The basic rules were to "stay out of trouble" and to be home for dinner before the street lights came on. I usually managed the second, but not always the first. Dad had a "boys will be boys" attitude as long as I did not challenge his authority or fail to get the lawn mowed on schedule. I do not think he worried much about me because he had an adventuresome childhood himself, growing up on farms and ranches. Mom, on the other hand, would have been upset if she knew all that I was up to—so I usually did not tell her. If asked about my activities, a few details might be judiciously omitted.

In the summer and on weekends, I often rode the mile to our elementary school where a game of baseball ("over the line"), basketball, or tackle football usually awaited. When a large group of us gathered, "hide and seek" and "tag" were also favorites. It was better that my Mom did not know that we had discovered a "secret" way to climb onto the roof of the school buildings as part of these games. We would run and jump on the tops of classrooms and hallways to escape being "tagged." Many days ended with me racing home when I finally noticed that the streetlights had come on.

Another favorite pastime was war. As children growing up in the 1950s, we saw countless movies about World War II on television. We imitated them by building forts and doing battle. It would often begin with sticks for guns and complicated rules about what you were supposed to do when you were "shot."

Our play often escalated to throwing dirt clods and rocks when the "rules of war" were broken. Battles ended when one group accused the other of not playing fair, or more often, when someone was hit by an incoming projectile and began crying.

When I wasn't playing a game for the "world championship" or fighting "epic" battles against the Germans, I loved to explore the open spaces that still surrounded our tract. One day as I walked through an orange grove that spread east of our house, I came upon a clearing with some dilapidated buildings. Scattered among them, partially swallowed by tall weeds, was a collection of rusted machinery and long pipes. It all held great fascination for a young explorer. To top it off, in the middle of the clearing, standing several stories tall like a monolith, was an abandoned oil derrick. I could not believe my eyes. To a boy who had not yet turned ten, this was the greatest discovery of all time. I could not wait to bring my friends to see it. My status rose as I took small groups to view the colossus.

As my discovery, I claimed the right to set the rules at the site. I decided which boys were allowed to test themselves by climbing up the angled wooden beams of the fifty-foot tower. I also determined which of the massive valves on the derrick were "safe" to rotate and which were "too dangerous."

The square derrick platform was over twenty feet on a side and ranged from five to ten feet above the surrounding ground. Our imaginations could transform this stage into a sea-tossed sailing vessel, a battleship under enemy attack, or a fortress protected by all manner of exotic weaponry.

Hanging down to the platform from the wooden tower was a wire cable. We transformed it into a giant swing by fashioning a loop at its end. We would run across the platform with the cable in our hands and jump on with our feet at the last moment, hanging on for dear life as it swung slowly through space beyond the edge. It was exhilarating to glide through the air like "Tarzan of the Jungle" for twenty or twenty-five feet. For a split second at the apex, we would be suspended high above the debris below.

Mom never heard about the oil derrick.

I know I lived a fortunate childhood. I escaped with more pleasant memories than scars. For this, I am sincerely grateful.

-- What were your adventures in childhood?
-- How might you add to someone else's childhood memories? (perhaps a grandchild?)

Nostalgia Food

I like burnt toast—and I know why.

Sometime while I was in elementary school, my dad bought a new toaster. I'm sure it was the latest technology. When you put the bread in, the slice would slowly lower as the toaster elements turned bright red. When the toast was done (according to the setting you selected), there would be an audible click. Slowly the toast would rise as the elements cooled. It was genius.

Dad was the toast master. His chair was next to the gleaming chrome appliance that sat on the side counter of our kitchenette. Watching him use the toaster was like watching a magic act. I begged to insert the bread—to be the sorcerer's apprentice. Having toaster privileges was a great honor.

Like people, as the toaster aged it developed some quirks. The lowering mechanism would only accept the bread if it had the correct mass and velocity upon insertion. Getting the toaster to lower the bread took just the right flick of the wrist—not too hard, not too light. Multiple attempts were the rule. Success on the first try was occasion for celebration.

At the other end of the process, the release timing became less precise. Sometimes the toaster would raise the bread up after barely warming it. This would necessitate reinsertion. The toaster would then become even more selective. When my dad attempted and failed on multiple tries, I learned some new vocabulary.

141

Most often, the toast emerged as a slice of smoking charcoal. The toaster setting was now irrelevant. So Dad developed a countermeasure. At the first smell of burning toast, he would wop the side of the toaster with the back of his hand. Apparently stunned, the toaster would release the toast—slightly burned but still edible.

We had that toaster for over a decade. There was never a discussion of replacing it. Raised in the Great Depression, my parents had learned to make do with what they had. We adapted.

And that is how I learned to like burnt toast.

Certain foods are connected to memories. For example, when I am sick, I crave the comfort of chicken noodle soup. And I don't mean some homemade secret family recipe. I mean standard, cheap, Andy Warhol, Campbell's chicken noodle soup. The kind where you eat the five tiny pieces of chicken meat you find, hunt down the buttery noodles until they are all gone, and then throw out most of the salty broth. For me, it remains a magic elixir.

And don't get me started about Thanksgiving. On the Holidays, I want sweet memories, not culinary adventures. Bring out some chestnut-horseradish stuffing that you saw demonstrated on TV and I am gone. Try your experimental recipes on your own time. I want my nostalgia food, please.

-- What are your nostalgia foods?
-- What memories are attached to them?

Best Friends

I went through a series of best friends in elementary and high school. Relationships waxed and waned—a natural progression as interests changed.

Les was tall like me and shared my love of basketball. We shot "horse" and played "one-on-one" constantly. We were both thrilled to make the fifth-grade team.

One day, Les almost got us killed. We were at his house when his mom was not home. He wanted to start the BBQ to cook us some hot dogs. We were hungry and the charcoal was not catching fast enough, so Les decided to pour some lighter fluid on it. The stream of fluid caught fire and the flames dashed all the way up to the can. Fortunately for our young faces, it did not explode.

Les's mom was divorced, so I learned that not all families were like mine. He struggled with the absence of his father.

I continued to grow tall through intermediate school while he did not. When Les was cut from the high school basketball team, our friendship cooled for the last time. Our bond of common interest was broken.

In sixth grade, I went through a short phase when Billy was my best friend. We sat next to each other in class and sometimes walked home together.

His dad was an engineer of some kind whose garage was full of cool electronic stuff. When Billy took me on a tour one day, it sparked my curiosity. He loaned me some books on electricity and electromagnetism that his dad had bought for him.

Billy was very bright and he became my science mentor. We even built a small transistor radio together (which picked up two or three stations). Billy did not like sports—my favorite pastime—so it was difficult to sustain our friendship for more than a few months. Nevertheless, I probably have Billy to thank for the fact that I became a science teacher.

My best friend for a while in seventh grade was Steve. He knew where his father hid Playboy magazines. Steve also contributed to my education.

Peter was my friend in eighth grade. He was super nice, smart, and a favorite with both students and teachers. He was a "good kid" and part of the popular crowd. He was elected student body president and spoke at eighth-grade graduation.

As a freshman in high school, Peter completely changed. He hung out with the "tough" kids, started smoking, and got into trouble at school. I never figured out what happened to change him so dramatically. We never talked about it. Although he later got back on track, we were never close again. We had taken our own paths—in different directions.

When I first entered high school, I was painfully shy— one of those kids who often ate lunch alone. I noticed another boy who ate alone. One day I sat down next to him. His name was Matt.

It did not take me long to discover why Matt had few friends. He was obsessed with monsters and horror movies. His bedroom was crammed with monster comic books and his walls were covered with horror movie posters. I didn't share his passion.

Matt almost turned me to a life of crime. We were in Sav-on Drug Store when he told me he wanted to steal some decals out of the model airplane boxes. I don't think he really needed the decals. I think he just wanted to steal something. Against my anxiety and better judgment, I became his accomplice. We opened boxes and stuffed the decals in our pockets. (Remember when store items were not hermetically sealed in impenetrable plastic?) When he hid a complete model airplane box under his jacket, I walked out in fearful protest. Once clear of the store, I happily gave him the evidence of our crime. I fully expected to hear police sirens as I hurried home with a guilty conscience.

This episode put an abrupt end to our friendship.

Each of my childhood friends was unique. Each taught me lessons about the world or myself.

I have also had friendships that reached a different depth and have lasted for decades. Also born of common interest in high school, graduate school, or church, these relationships have continued to grow in trust and emotional intimacy. We have shared ourselves openly and supported each other through the challenges of life. I am grateful to have been so blessed.

For example, my high school friend Carolyn is now my wife—and my high school friend Grant married us!

-- What did you learn from your best friends in school?
-- What memories of friends are worth revisiting?
-- Are there some old friends you want to reconnect with?

I Am Grateful

I am grateful I have known true love.

I am grateful I became a teacher.

I am grateful to be alive and healthy.

I am grateful to live in freedom.

I am grateful for my parents.

I am grateful for my children.

I am grateful for good friends.

I am grateful for my education.

I am grateful for my home and neighborhood.

I am grateful for the beauty of nature.

I am grateful for my spiritual awareness.

I am grateful for the pleasures of food and sex (sorry kids).

I am grateful for my athletic ability.

I am grateful for my intelligence.

I am grateful for my modesty.

I am grateful for my sense of humor.

-- What are you grateful for?

Basketball Rules

As a new high school without any seniors, our varsity basketball team had lost every league game the previous season. Our cross-town rival Sierra High had embarrassed us twice: 61-37 and 58-39.

With all of our starters returning, there were high expectations for the new season, but by the time we faced Sierra, our record was a disappointing 9 wins and 8 losses. Sierra, by contrast, had only lost once in the new season—and was favored to repeat as league champs.

Sierra started several experienced seniors. As we warmed up, I could just feel their "cockiness" as they ran their layup drill at the opposite end of their home court. Only a sophomore, it was my first year on varsity. I had never played in a rivalry game like this and my mouth was dry with nerves.

The gym was absolutely packed. Each school's cheerleaders took turns exhorting their fans to scream louder than the other side. In 1962, it was still cool to yell for your team.

When the game began, it was as if a year's worth of pent-up frustration was released. To our own amazement, we stormed to an 18-9 lead in the first quarter. Sierra, however, came fighting back. By the time we started the fourth quarter, our lead was only 4 points. Both teams began exchanging baskets and scoring at an astonishing rate, racking up a total of forty-one points in those last eight minutes. The gym was so loud it actually hurt my ears and with each score, the crowd got more deafening.

At some point in this last quarter, I entered a trance-like state that athletes sometimes describe as "being in the zone." I no longer heard the crowd, I didn't feel tired, and my body was moving and reacting as if it was not under my conscious control. I was totally focused.

We had a one-point lead with less than a minute to play. Sierra had the ball and passed it around until it came to the guy I was guarding. As a natural center playing forward, it was still uncomfortable for me to defend away from the basket. The senior I was matched-up against was one of their better players—and much quicker than me. With seconds ticking away, we were isolated on the right side of the court. He turned and we stood face-to-face.

At this point, everything went into slow motion. He faked to my right and then tried to dribble around me to my left. In a surreal moment that I can still remember vividly, my body moved—seemingly without my commanding it—back and to the left to cut him off at the baseline. He knocked me down and the whistle blew. For a split second, everybody froze as we looked at the referee. Then, with an exaggerated motion, he called an offensive foul against Sierra and gave us the ball out of bounds.

The crowd went crazy. My normally reserved coach jumped in the air and started clapping wildly. I knew then that all of those exhausting defensive drills had paid off.

The drama, however, was not over.

As we tried to run out the clock, Sierra's star player stole the ball. We fouled him with only two seconds left in the game. He would shoot free throws.

We still had a one point lead, but the penalty was one and one. If he made the first free throw, the game would be tied and he would be awarded a second shot. If he made both, they would win.

He was shooting over eighty percent from the line for the season, so our defeat seemed assured.

His critical first free throw went up, bounced slowly around the rim—and then fell off.

The Sierra center and I both went high for the rebound. I managed to grab it and pull it away from him. The buzzer sounded and the game was over. We had defeated mighty Sierra 54-53.

-- Can you remember a "peak experience?" Perhaps it wasn't in sports, but a music recital, play, art show, or drag race. Did you sell the most Girl Scout Cookies or build the fastest Pinewood Derby car? Did you get the highest grade on an English essay or class project?

-- How could you acknowledge others (family members, friends, children, or youth) to help them have the exhilarating feelings that come with well-deserved praise and recognition?

Nightmare on Elm Avenue

I was watching football on a lazy fall Saturday during my junior year of high school. I didn't pay much attention when Mom answered the phone. "Yes, he is right here," I heard her say. I sat up and gave her a puzzled look. She covered the mouthpiece with her hand and—without making a sound—mouthed the words, "It's a girl from school."

I didn't talk to girls in person, much less on the phone. My heart was already racing with nervousness as Mom passed me the handset.

"Hello?" I said with puzzlement in my voice.

"This is Jennifer Rollins," she began. "Do you remember me from school?"

I had no clue.

"Sure, how are you?" I didn't want to hurt her feelings. My mind raced through all the Jennifers I knew. I decided it must be that girl from my chemistry class.

"Has anyone invited you to the Winter Formal?" she asked.

Winter Formal at our school was a girl ask guy dance. I had zero interest in attending *any* dance. It had not even crossed my mind.

"No," I replied.

"My friend is going with Ken Stevens and I was hoping we could double date."

Ken was a great guy and good friend. (He was voted Student Body President our senior year.) I thought, the girls must be O.K if he said yes. I also remembered that Jennifer from chemistry was friendly—and good looking.

Before I could think any further, I heard myself say, "Sure, I'd love to to."

"Great. Let's all meet in front of the snack bar during break to talk about details," she continued.

"I'll be there," I replied.

"Bye."

That was it. I was going to Winter Formal with that nice girl from my chemistry class.

Monday morning I found Ken during nutrition break. "Do you know these girls?" I asked.

The look on Ken's face worried me. He said, "I think they are sophomores. I thought *you* knew them. Betty told me you said yes to Jennifer, so I figured it was O.K." We both smiled in recognition of how we had been trapped.

Two girls approached—and neither one was Jennifer from chemistry. Ken and I shared an "Uh-oh, what have we done?" glance before one of them started to speak.

"Hi, I'm Jennifer and this is Betty."

By my junior year, I was 6' 7" and thin as a shadow. From my vantage point, Jennifer and Betty looked like they were about 4' tall. They were both plain and a little overweight. I don't like to be unkind, so let's just say that puberty had not yet worked its magic on them. If I had given them nicknames, I would have called them Frumpy and Dumpy.

Jennifer continued her well rehearsed presentation. "We want to go to Steak and Stein for dinner before the dance. My dress is pink and Betty's is powder blue so you can match our corsages. You can pick me up at 6:00 and then we will pick up Ken and Betty." She finished her litany with, "You will have to rent tuxedoes you know."

Ken and I were speechless. After the girls walked away, we laughed and decided that we would be good sports and try to make the best of it.

Mom's car was a nine year old blue Dodge sedan. Its best days were well behind it. I was not allowed to drive Dad's car yet and certainly no one from our neighborhood was going to rent a limosine. The old blue Dodge would have to do.

I used paint restorer on the dull finish and waxed the refreshed paint to a nice shine. There was little I could do with the shabby, nicotine stained interior. I decided I could at least repair the holes in the side panels next to the arm rest. As an "improvement," I cut my blue dress socks into patches and sewed them over the holes. It looked as ridiculous as it sounds.

After Mom and I managed to get me dressed in my tux, I was off to pick up Jennifer. I turned on Elm Avenue and started looking at house numbers. Then *bang*, a tire blew.

I walked down to Jennifer's house to tell her I would be late. I knew I had a spare tire and tools in the trunk. After meeting Jennifer's parents and explaining the situation to them, Jennifer's father insisted that he would change the tire for me. He would not allow me to damage my rented tuxedo. I was mortified as I stood watching him put on the spare.

We finally made it to Steak and Stein, one of the "special occasion" restaurants in town. As we were being seated, Jennifer insisted that she and Betty sit on the same side of the booth. We later realized the motive. They spent the whole evening whispering and giggling back and forth to each other. It was as if Ken and I were not there.

Both girls ordered the most expensive steak on the menu. (Even though it was girl ask guy, the guys were expected to pay.) They hardly touched their food because they were so busy talking. When it was time to leave, they asked for "doggie bags." Ken and I just looked at each other in disbelief.

The strange behavior continued at the dance. The girls spent the whole night giggling and making trips to the bathroom. I don't remember if we even danced.

Any anxiety I had about whether I needed to kiss her good night at the front door turned out to be wasted energy. Jennifer marched straight into her house with barely a good-bye.

I hope the evening was all that Jennifer expected. She never really said. (I don't think we interacted again the entire time we were both in school together.)

Two weeks later I accidently discovered two "doggie bags" of moldy steak stuffed under the back seat of the blue Dodge.

What an experience.

-- What awkward or embarrassing moments from your youth are still lodged in your memory after all these years?

Senior Sock Hop

Several senior women ("blue hairs?") formed a circle on the dance floor of our community ballroom. After half a century, the familiar rock and roll that the DJ played still had hypnotic power over them. (Their balding husbands choose to stay at the tables and drink another glass of wine.)

The ladies' bodies were a little thicker, their joints a little stiffer, but if you squinted your eyes nearly shut and opened your imagination, you could see 17-year-old girls at their high school sock hop. The carefully choreographed moves were still there, copied from American Bandstand and practiced for hours in front of the bedroom mirror.

The glow on the faces said that their minds were back in that sparsely decorated gym, reliving teenage triumphs. The flirty eyes, the coy smiles, the sexy moves—as suggestive as good girls were allowed to display in those self-conscious days. It was all automatic—muscle memory re-engaged after decades of working, raising families, and growing older. For just a few minutes, it was an uninhibited expression of youth recaptured.

Watching them brought an odd range of emotions. My initial mix of nostalgia and melancholy was quickly overwhelmed by pure appreciation and joy. In all their lumpy, saggy, movement restricted glory, how beautiful they were.

-- What are your favorite memories from high school?
-- What would you tell your grandchildren about the trials of being a teenager "back in the day?"

154

Becoming a Man

When did I first feel like a man?

There are the obvious answers. One might think my honeymoon night would qualify. After all, I was still a virgin. But no. If I am honest, that was pretty much a disaster. Ignorance is not always bliss.

Another good choice might be the day my first child was born. I don't know if I have ever felt such a high. Eventually, the euphoria was replaced by a sobering sense of responsibility. Supporting, protecting, and nurturing my children is a core part of my definition of manhood for sure. But some earlier, less obvious moments also come to mind.

One involves Bill—father-in-law from my first marriage. He was a solid, hard-working man of character and integrity. He lived his Midwest values and I respected him greatly for that.

It was the first Christmas my wife and I celebrated in our newly purchased home. Usually, presents from my in-laws came with two names on them, but this one just said, "To Wayne, From Bill." I unwrapped the package to find a top-of-the-line Craftsman hammer from Sears. It had a black grip, a beautiful ivory colored neck, and gleaming steel head. Bill simply said, "You're going to be needing that around here."

It was a thoughtful gift, but to me, it meant much more than might be obvious. I felt that Bill was saying to me "A man needs good tools. Welcome to the club."

I still have that hammer—in the toolbox that he also gave to me that Christmas. I think of Bill every time I wrap my hand around the handle, now scarred and discolored from decades of use (both my hand and the hammer). My eyes can still moisten as I think of his gift of acknowledgment that made me feel like a man.

Another milestone on my way to manhood occurred even earlier. I was fifteen years old when my Dad took me out for my first driving lesson. We found some recently paved roads in a still vacant subdivision. It was such a milestone for me that I can still recall how the car smelled as I got behind the wheel for the first time.

Our family car was a column shift Dodge. It took a while for me to begin to get a feel for using the clutch. Dad was surprisingly patient. Soon my confidence began to soar as I got the hang of it—until I slowed to take a corner and the car began to lug. "Don't forget to downshift," Dad calmly instructed.

When I felt that the lesson was about over, Dad surprised me by saying, "Why don't you drive us home." That felt like a remarkable validation.

As we made our way down the "real" streets, Dad noticed that I was going well under the posted speed limit. "Unless a cop is right on your tail," he confided, "you can safely go 5 miles per hour over the speed limit."

The sharing of that "secret knowledge" by my father felt like my initiation to manhood.

-- When did you first feel like a "real" woman or man?

156

Television

We are the television generation. We followed the radio generation and preceded the internet generation and smartphone generation. Each successive generation may be defined by its dominant technology.

As a child in the early 1950s, I loved *Howdy Doody*. My friends and I would gather after school to watch on our tiny black and white TV. In 1956, the show moved to Saturday mornings. I watched alone then because— as a 9-year-old—I didn't want my friends to know I still liked the silly show.

It was an age of innocence. No tabloid journalism to divulge what was really going on when Howdy Doody failed to appear on the show for several days. We were told that Howdy was traveling the country "following the national election campaign." In reality, the puppeteer had taken Howdy off the set because of a contract dispute with "Buffalo Bob" Smith—the show's creator. The dispute was resolved when Smith had a replacement Howdy built. It maintained the 48 freckles—one for each state—but now had more handsome features. To explain the change, we viewers were told that Howdy had decided to have plastic surgery. (Seriously)

We never had more than one television in our home. Dad and Mom were in charge of program selection. My brother and I were allowed to respectfully express an opinion, but whining was not tolerated. If we didn't like the program they selected, we could go to our room and play. (I often walked out on Liberace.) But usually, we watched TV as a family—a shared experience that I remember fondly.

157

With only three major networks, a good portion of the country was also having shared experiences. As a nation, we were informed by the news coverage of the Vietnam War overseas and civil rights confrontations in the South. Together we mourned the assassination of President Kennedy and stayed up late to watch men walk on the moon. In the 1970s, meetings and events were not scheduled on Monday nights because so many of us were watching football. After each episode of the Roots miniseries, the whole nation shared reactions "around the water cooler" the next day.

Then as now, there were divisive political differences in the country. Yet, somehow, our shared television experiences helped us feel more bonded as a nation. With fewer shared TV experiences today, it can feel like the country is more fractured. My choice of television news network might alienate me from my neighbor who chooses to watch a different channel. It can feel like we are The Divided States of America. (I felt clever writing this, but I am sure I am not the first.)

Early televisions were quirky, semi-reliable devices. If the picture was bad, Dad would first check the rooftop antenna. He had to point it in just the right direction to maximize the signal from the broadcast towers in the mountains above Los Angeles.

If that wasn't the problem, he would remove the pegboard from the back of the set to reveal a dozen or more glowing tubes. Using his previous experience (and some psychic powers), he would remove a handful of the tubes and take them to our neighborhood Sav-on Drug Store.

Next to the photo department (remember getting pictures developed?) was a "tube tester." Prongs on the tubes were matched with holes in the tester. Once inserted, Dad let me push a button that produced a display: green=good, yellow=weak, red=bad.

Finding either a good tube or bad tube was reason for celebration. A reading of yellow became an agonizing judgment call. The guessing game might require several frustrating trips to the store. If inserting the replacement tube back into our set at home did not solve the problem, Dad would explode with words like "Dag Nabbit!"—and then the investigation would calmly continue. He did not like to be defeated.

Remember when all channel changing, volume control, and set adjustment required hands-on-knob manipulation? We used the "TV Guide" page in the newspaper to select our shows. "Channel surfing" was unheard of because it was too much work.

Early televisions had a tendency to lose their vertical or horizontal "hold." For no apparent reason, the picture would start rolling, often starting slowly and then increasing speed. Alternately, sometimes the picture would collapse sideways into a mass of angled lines.

Correcting the issues required delicate adjustment of small knobs that on some TVs were inexplicably located on the back of the sets. This meant that adjustment required two people—one to adjust the knob and one to observe the result. If one was alone, it became a frustrating game of trial and error.

Eventually, the manufacturers hid the controls behind a flip down door in the front of the set. Even then, adjustment might not be easy. If the picture was rolling down, for example, the slightest turn of the control might reverse the rolling in the opposite direction. It could take a safe cracker's fingertip sensitivity to find the perfect balance to get the picture to stay still.

My Dad liked westerns. As a boy, he had read every western themed book in his small-town Kansas library. Zane Grey was his favorite author.

Fortunately for my Dad, westerns were some of the most popular television shows in the '50s and '60s. We watched *a lot* of westerns, including *Gunsmoke* starring James Arness, *Bonanza* with Lorne Greene and Michael Landon, and *Maverick* starring James Garner. I also remember *Have Gun, Will Travel*, *The Rifleman*, and *The Lone Ranger*. It was always clear who the good guys were. You could rest assured that justice would triumph in the end.

We also watched a lot of comedy and variety shows. I was introduced to the masters—Red Skelton, Jack Benny, Burns and Allen. And of course, Bob Hope. We waited for his specials with anticipation. His monologues were funny even to a young kid who didn't follow politics or understand double entendre. Some of our biggest laughs came from Allen Funt's *Candid Camera* and Art Linkletter's *People are Funny*.

My parents enjoyed music shows. The corny schmaltz of Lawrence Welk might push me back into my room to listen to Vin Scully announce a Dodger game. Perry Como was bearable; although he seemed so relaxed, I worried that he might fall off his stool at any moment.

Everyone watched *Ed Sullivan* on Sunday nights. It was a true variety show with music, magic, comedians, jugglers, and circus acts. After 1957, we usually only watched half of the show because the first half conflicted with *Maverick*. An exception was made for three consecutive Sundays in February 1964—for the Beatles. My dad said someone must have put a bowl on the Beatles' heads when they got their haircut. I don't think my parents ever really got the Fab Four.

My brother and I had to get our baths immediately after dinner on Sunday night so that we didn't miss our favorite programs. No DVR to delay the program to our own time schedule. No On-Demand reruns or streaming video to catch up on a missed show. No pause button to stop a show in mid-presentation. What a different world we live in now.

A favorite show for many years was Disney. It changed names and nights several times—*Walt Disney's Disneyland* (1954-1958), *Walt Disney Presents* (1958-1961), *Walt Disney's Wonderful World of Color* (1961-1969), and onward.

What marketing genius. Essentially, the program has been a decades-long infomercial for Disney Theme Parks and Disney Movies. Beginning in the fall of 1954, every episode of the show contained "making of Disneyland" segments and teasers, creating unprecedented demand by the time the park actually opened in July of 1955.

Television was not the center of our lives when I was growing up. It was rarely on in the daytime except for weekend sports. If one of our favorite shows was not on, the TV stayed off. We were just as happy playing cards or board games like *Monopoly* or *Clue*. The entertainment provided by television seemed to be in balance with other aspects of our family life.

After I left home to attend college, some television programs took on an edgier tone—reflecting a changing culture. From 1967-1969 (when they lost their battle with the network censors), *The Smothers Brothers Comedy Hour* was groundbreaking. I loved it when their jokes were so counter-culture cool that I knew my parents would not understand them. In 1968, *Rowan & Martin's Laugh-in* imbedded serious political commentary into such a silly slapstick format that it anesthetized the antiestablishment bite. Can you imagine dour Richard Nixon saying "Sock it to me?" I am sure he (like my parents) never understood that the phrase could have a sexual connotation.

Despite predictable plots and dialogue, I loved the *Mod Squad* (1968-1973). They were the hippest cops on TV—a longhaired rebel rejecting his wealthy parents; an afro-sporting Watts riot survivor; and a golden-haired hippy girl runaway. The show had everything that was cool.

Mary Tyler Moore—for the first time on television (1970)—provided an example of a never-married, strong, independent professional woman. *All in the Family* (1971) and *Mash* (1972) drove nails into the coffins of condoned bigotry and the Vietnam War.

It is interesting that the most influential programs were usually comedies. At its best, television managed to catch our attention with humor, and then enlighten us without our knowing it.

-- What are your favorite TV memories?
-- What associations do you have with the word "Disney?"
-- How did television open your mind?

A Game of Takeaway # 2

When I recall my family memories, my smile of appreciation is often followed by a moment of sadness. No one in my nuclear family is still alive. All the memories are mine alone.

I remember decades ago when I would join my parents and brother for holidays or birthdays, the conversation would invariably turn to shared memories. Remember that Christmas when Dad's gift to Mom was a nylon stocking filled with money? Remember when we drove across the desert on our way to Kansas with no air conditioning—just that dry ice cooler in the window? Remember the fishing trip to Convict Lake when we drove that scary one lane road carved into the cliff?

My memories are still vivid, but I miss being able to reminisce with my family.

Many of us have already lost one or both parents. Others will have the experience in the coming years. It can hit hard when you realize that you have become the matriarch or patriarch of the family—the next in line.

I recently spoke with an 89-year-old neighbor. She seemed a little quiet so I asked her what was going on. She said that she had been to a memorial service that morning. "All of my old friends and most of my family have died. It is the hardest thing about getting old. If you live long enough, you end up feeling very alone." Coming from a woman who is normally positive and upbeat, the statement gave me pause.

We have all experienced the unexpected passing of friends or loved ones, but as we approach our eighties and beyond, there will be a crescendo of loss. We will need the support of our religion or personal philosophy. We will need to rely on each other as sources of comfort and strength. Shared pain is less debilitating.

We are the first generation to have regular visitors to our home that we don't actually know. They entered via television. Some TV personalities began to feel like family.

My father liked to watch the evening news, so I became friends with Chet Huntley and David Brinkley. Later, Tom Brokaw became a regular visitor. For other families, Walter Cronkite and Dan Rather were invited guests. From 1983 to 2005, I developed a relationship with Peter Jennings. When he was taken by cancer, it felt like a personal loss.

Actors in weekly dramas and comedies, soap opera stars, and talk show hosts all could provide the comfort of familiarity. We even let Johnny Carson into our bedrooms!

When our TV family members have their shows canceled or they retire, we miss them. Imagine our feelings when we eventually hear that they have moved on to the ultimate stage. Our hearts will mourn as if we actually knew them. The truth is, we will be mourning the passing of part of our own lives.

I remember experiencing an emptiness when I heard that John Denver had died. He was a hero to me in the 1970s as both a performer and environmental activist. We sang along to his music on family trips to Yosemite, Yellowstone, Glacier, and Rocky Mountain National Parks. He crashed his experimental aircraft in 1997 at the age of fifty-three.

I was also moved by the deaths of John Lennon in 1980 at the age of forty and Michael Jackson in 2009 at the age of fifty.

Recently, two music icons passed in quick succession. For several days, the media reminded us how much Boomers Glenn Frey (Eagles) and David Bowie added to the soundtrack of our lives. Their deaths felt different. They did not die of an accident, overdose, or assassination like previous icons. Instead, they died of disease. They died because their bodies let them down. They died because they were...about my age.

That hit home—in a scary way.

It will not be long until such losses will be a weekly occurrence. I am not going to like that. It will be like looking through the photo album of my life and watching treasured pictures fade away one by one.

For us Older Boomers, it will hit hardest when Paul McCartney and Mick Jagger go. Bob Dylan, Stevie Wonder, and Brian Wilson will also leave a mark. For Younger Boomers, Prince was a milestone loss. For others, the departure of Madonna, Sting, or Bono may give pause.

Of course, the impact of each celebrity death will depend on our age, music tastes, TV viewing habits, favorite movies, and sports preferences. Some stars have touched us more than others.

One that may hit me hard is Kareem Abdul-Jabbar (if he goes first). We are the same age. As Lou Alcindor, he dominated college basketball at UCLA as I watched with awe from the bench at Stanford.

In my sophomore season, we played in Pauley Pavilion on the UCLA campus. Toward the end of the game, the Bruins had nearly doubled our score and coach put me in as a "white flag of surrender." I managed to foul Alcindor before John Wooden had the chance to take him out. Kareem would have no memory of this event, but it was the highpoint of my college career.

It hardly seems fair. As we cope with the physical takeaways of aging, we are hit with the emotional takeaways on top of it. As Bette Davis said, "Getting old is not for sissies."

Acceptance is going to be hard work.

Two additional thoughts about loss:

1) *Leave no regrets.* Spend time with the people you love. Let them know how you feel about them. Savor the sharing, laughing, and reminiscing while you can.

2) *It is O.K. to feel.* Pain and sorrow are the price we pay for loving and caring. Recovery and acceptance come faster when we allow ourselves to be human and experience our emotions.

-- Who can you share your feelings with to lighten your burden?
-- How can you be there for others in their time of grieving?.

The Cold War

War! Huh – Good God y'all
What is it good for?
Absolutely nothing   *-Edwin Starr*

We grew up in wartime. The "hot wars" in Korea and Vietnam were extensions of the Cold War that began after WWII and lasted over four decades. It was different from any previous war. Both sides had intercontinental ballistic missiles tipped with nuclear warheads. The vast Atlantic and Pacific no longer provided us with a protected homeland.

Do you remember practicing "duck and cover" drills in elementary school? We heard the air raid siren tested every Friday at noon. We watched films that showed the melting of mannequins and the disintegration of buildings resulting from a nuclear blast. Even as an elementary school child, I realized that if a nuclear bomb went off anywhere close, crawling under my school desk would be absurdly useless. I would be completely incinerated—along with my desk.

Remember the signs posted on big buildings that led to bomb shelters? Remember the newspaper diagrams showing concentric rings of destruction from a Russian nuclear bomb blast? Our house was always inside the rings.

All of this was deeply disturbing to me. I felt scared. It wasn't the horror movie kind of scared, but just a constant low-level fear. I could not understand how the leaders of the world could let things get so out of hand. I felt vulnerable to the whims of madmen. Sometimes I wished Dad would build a home bomb shelter as some people did during those years.

167

From time to time, events in the news would increase my level of fear. One morning in the fall of 1956 (age nine) I was watching the news on TV when I heard the reporters talking about the "Crisis in Suez." Essentially Egypt and Britain were fighting over the right to control shipping through the vital Suez Canal. Russia was backing Egypt and the newscasters described the events as a "showdown between East and West" which could lead to nuclear confrontation. Although there was never any real threat of nuclear war, the way the newscasters exaggerated the conflict produced a fear in me that I clearly remember to this day.

In 1957, Russia launched the first satellite, Sputnik. Just after dark, our whole family stood in the backyard and watched the tiny speck of light move across the sky. The TV played recordings of the constant "pinging" sound that it broadcast as it traveled through space. We now know that it carried no weapons, but everything the Russians did was threatening because we knew they were out to destroy us. I remember how vulnerable I felt realizing that Sputnik passed over my house every 101 minutes—and nothing could be done about it.

The most serious threat to the United States was the Cuban Missile Crisis of October, 1962. The Russians had placed missiles in Cuba with the ability to launch nuclear warheads into the U.S. President Kennedy threatened to invade Cuba to destroy the missiles and Soviet Premier Khrushchev threatened war in retaliation. Both men seemed locked into their positions with no way to avoid conflict. The U.S. loaded nuclear weapons on its bombers and went to military alert level DEFCON2 (nuclear war is imminent) for the first time in history.

News reports followed the escalating tensions step-by-step as we moved to the brink of nuclear war. At fifteen, I was old enough to understand what was happening—and to realize that my parents could not protect me from this kind of insanity.

The Cuban Missile Crisis was resolved in the 11th hour by secret negotiations. The Russians removed the missiles in exchange for a public pledge by the U.S. not to invade Cuba—and a private pledge to remove similar short-range missiles near the Soviet border in Turkey. The avoidance of all-out war, however, did not remove the damage to my sense of security.

Even when there was no political crisis in the news, we all knew that we were one mechanical malfunction or one human error away from nuclear annihilation. We tried to laugh at it in movies like *Dr. Strangelove or, How I Learned to Stop Worrying and Love the Bomb*. The movie was darkly funny. Nuclear war was not funny.

The Cold War left unseen psychological casualties—and I was at least one of the wounded.

-- How were you affected by the cold war?

The Vietnam War

During the Cold War, communism was perceived to be like a cancer. It was commonly thought that if its spread was not stopped, it would destroy the entire free world. In the early 1950s, we fought to stop it from spreading down the Korean Peninsula. Vietnam was seen as a similar "domino" ready to fall in the early 1960s.

Although the war started in 1959, President Johnson began escalating United States involvement in 1963. Eventually, the "Vietnam Conflict" (it was never a declared war) became the longest and most expensive war in our history up to that point. (We used more munitions than in all of WWII). Before it ended in 1975, it would change the direction of the country and fuel a cultural revolution.

For the older men of the Boomer generation, the military draft hung over our heads like the sharp blade of a guillotine. The draft moved the Vietnam War from an abstract political discussion to a highly personal, life changing issue. It was one thing to take two years out of your life to serve your country. It was quite another to risk your life in a war that many of us felt was unjust and irrational.

As U.S. troop deployments escalated in the late '60s, so did the grim statistics of dead and wounded that were graphically displayed on the television news each night. Younger people who have grown up in the era of the "all volunteer" army may find it difficult to comprehend the dread associated with *Selective Service*.

Most of us Older Boomer men have a story to tell about their experiences with the Draft. My first year at Stanford I was given a "student deferment," a postponement of being drafted that was commonly granted. As military needs grew, those deferments were canceled. I was then granted a "marriage deferment." (I was married at the beginning of my junior year.) Soon those were canceled. Then I was granted a deferment for being too tall. (6'6" was the limit.) They raised the limit to 6'8". After running out of options and appeals, I received notification that I was classified "1-A" and could be drafted into military service at any time. Like many of my friends, I tried to make jokes and feign an air of resignation, but underneath I alternately felt frustration, anger, anxiety, and despair.

I did not want to go to war, especially this war. Some students considered going to Canada to escape the Draft, but I was a married man—not to mention that I did not want to spend the rest of my life as a fugitive from justice. I looked into the Navy and Air Force officer programs, which I thought might be safer, but there were waiting lists and the commitment time was five or six years. Finally, I went to the Army recruiting office in San Jose. The advertised benefit of enlistment for college students was that I could pick a field for military training that related to my academic major. Perhaps, I thought, I could at least avoid the infantry where the casualty rate was highest.

I entered an office where a recruiting sergeant sat behind the desk in his pressed brown uniform and "spit-shined" shoes. He made an effort to be friendly and soon asked me what my major was in college. I told him "psychology."

171

He confidently opened a large book on his desk and said, "I'm sure we can find something related to that." He silently thumbed through the pages for a long time until a clear look of concern deepened on his face. I began to worry and sat forward to look at the book upside down from my side of the desk. He was looking for psychology under the alphabetical listings for "S." I was dumbfounded. I told him not to worry about it and hastily excused myself from his office. I knew I would not do well in this man's Army.

It seemed as if I had no good options. The frustration was maddening. Government leaders had repeatedly made poor decisions to get us deeper and deeper into this war and my life was going to be ruined—or ended—because of their hubris.

Finally, in late 1969, there was a ray of hope. The government announced that it would hold a "draft lottery." There was widespread belief that some draft boards were giving favorable treatment to the well connected. The lottery would randomly select birthdays from the calendar and assign them numbers from 1-366. Because of the projected manpower needs of the military, it was thought that only those who received a number below 230 would likely be drafted.

The day after the lottery was held, *The Stanford Daily* reported the following: "Stanford University held its breath for two hours last night as the first draft lottery since World War II decided the military fate of 8,000 Stanford students. Apprehension was great before the draw began and as birth dates were drawn, joy, despair, and confusion flowed freely across campus."

The lottery was held on December 1, 1969. I listened anxiously to the radio broadcast as the numbers were chosen in Washington DC. Tension and relief alternated as each birthday was drawn from a fishbowl and read to the nation. It was like life and death bingo. I held my breath between each announcement.

My heart lifted as the numbers passed 230. It sang for joy when my birthday was assigned a lottery number over 275. I would not be drafted. I could go on with my life. I would be able to complete graduate school and start my teaching career.

We were all affected by the Vietnam War. I felt fortunate that I did not have to actively participate. To those of you who did, I honor your service and sacrifice. I also mourn your losses, which were many.

-- How were you and the people you love affected by the Vietnam War?

Offspring

Eighty-six percent of Boomers have children. Only seven percent think it was a mistake.

I was surprised when I read these statistics. With the choices our generation had for family planning, I might have guessed that more of us would have opted for the freedom and economic benefit of remaining childless. Apparently, the primordial drive to procreate is powerful. Even among the percentage that did not have children, over half wish they had.

Personally, despite all the travails and frustrations, helping to raise children was profoundly fulfilling.

Still, having adult children may require adjustments. The genetic shuffle guarantees our children will not be just like us. Nor will they be the same as their siblings. Like the branches of an oak, each child grows to a unique form.

For some of us, that form provides the opportunity for close friendship. Such compatibility is a great blessing. In other cases, our children grow disappointingly distant. The bonds of love and caring we felt holding our dependent baby do not always translate into the closeness we desire with adult children.

Grandchildren reawaken the hope, providing a "redo" of sorts. With short bursts of energy and without the distractions of career or homemaking, we can now nurture a child with our full attention.

Loving a grandchild—without the responsibility of parenting—is a sweet experience.

Hippies and Hot Tubs

It was a New Age. At least that was my idealistic hope as an Early Boomer. Our parents' generation had survived the Great Depression and defeated fascism. Unfortunately, the political climate that followed produced a cold war with the Soviet Union and a hot war with North Vietnam. Racial bigotry was tolerated and gender inequality accepted. Self-expression was quashed by a rigid set of cultural norms. Our generation thought we could do better.

Many of us believed that the key to world peace, interpersonal harmony, and individual freedom was personal growth. If we could free ourselves of our "hang-ups," we would be free to love others without inhibition—and change the world. Drugs like marijuana and LSD could help free our minds. Personal growth experiences like encounter groups and EST could liberate us from our inhibitions.

Admittedly, many who adopted the "hippy" lifestyle were more interested in "sex, drugs and rock-n-roll" than in saving the world. Personal growth was a good cover story for youthful hedonism. But there were some of us true believers. We took the "Human Potential Movement" seriously.

In the '60s, the mecca for serious personal growth and liberation was *Esalen*—a beautiful little strip of property on the Big Sur Coast of California with spectacular ocean views and natural hot springs. Nudity was the dress code around the ocean front pool and hot tubs, sexuality was freely expressed, and experimentation with drugs (though officially discouraged) was common.

My friend Gerry suggested that I take a workshop called "Experiencing Esalen"—designed to provide a sample of several different avenues of personal growth offered at *Esalen Institute* (official name). Gerry wanted to drive his Karmann Ghia (a small sports car made by Volkswagen) up the coast. It was hilarious to watch me fold my 6' 7" frame into the tiny car, but somehow I managed and we were off on our weekend road trip.

We arrived after dark on a Friday night. I felt disoriented as I found my way to the meeting room where my workshop had already begun. Sitting on the floor in a rough circle were eighteen or twenty people. They were a mixture of sexes, ages, and "types"—ranging from "long hair hippie" to "clean cut business." Some seemed very comfortable and relaxed in this atmosphere while others were clearly uncomfortable and tense. I tried to look like the former while inside I felt like the latter.

The group leader was a very large woman with long graying hair who obviously had overcome the "hang-up" of being concerned about her appearance. She didn't smile much and gave off the "vibe" that she had led this workshop a few too many times to be enthusiastic about it.

I was suffering from "Ghia lag" and was hoping that the large woman was about to clarify the weekend schedule and then send us off to get comfortable in our rustic rooms. Instead, she struggled to her feet and told us we were going for a walk. She said we should leave our shoes in the room because we would be barefoot. We were instructed to walk in total silence and "open up our senses."

My sense of vision was not much use in the pitch-black darkness outside. My other senses told me we were walking down a dirt path along the cliff above the ocean. In due course, the line of people in front of me entered a strange looking structure. It was lit by flickering candlelight and I noticed it felt very warm and humid inside. Then I noticed something else. Everyone was taking off his or her clothes.

Gerry had prepared me to expect the unexpected, but this still came as a bit of a shock. I took off my clothes and tried to act as if this was normal behavior for me. I suspected that we must be in the bathhouse where the hot mineral pools were located. Everyone was still moving in silence, so I didn't ask any questions. My suspicions were soon confirmed as we moved into a room with several large concrete tubs along a long wall. The other side of the room had a row of canvas curtains through which my "open senses" could hear the Pacific Ocean.

The first tub I came too was already crowded with six or seven nude bodies, anchored in one corner by the large leader lady. She motioned for me to get in and—against all logic—I squeezed my body into the already overcrowded mass of nakedness. This was certainly a test for my contact phobia, for no matter how I maneuvered my body, it was impossible not to be touching the wet skin of several other people. To my astonishment, even more people were invited into our tub. There was nothing left to do but surrender.

The water was hot and soothing, but it was impossible to move my body into a comfortable position. I became aware of the first rule of naked hot tub use—maintain eye contact. Somehow, it felt more respectful to look people in the eye than to allow them to see me scanning their exposed body.

Surprisingly it did not feel as sensual or sexy as I might have imagined. I tried to think of it as a spiritual experience— although a crowded one.

After we could no longer call ourselves strangers, we moved to tables where we took turns receiving group massage. It was amazing to feel the soft stroking of several hands over different areas of the body (still thinking spiritual). The air was thick with the sweetness of scented oil mingling with the slight sulfur smell of the hot tubs. Added to this was the background sound of the ocean surging in a slow rhythm onto the rocks below. It was a delightful sensory overload.

Massaging others brought out surprising feelings of caring and connection. I did not know any of them as individuals, but I felt like I knew all of them in their unprotected humanity. I fell into a trance-like state with no awareness of time.

I was still feeling a wonderful combination of inner peace and emotional high when I later searched for my cabin. I entered to find Gerry sleeping soundly despite loud snoring from a man in another bed. The empty bunk looked uncomfortably short and incompatible with my current state of bliss, so I grabbed a blanket and walked to a grassy area near the pool. I wanted to enjoy the awesome beauty of the star-filled sky, but quickly fell asleep on the ground instead.

The next afternoon, some community members and workshop participants gathered for Esalen's version of a dance. We all took off our shoes (not our clothes) as we entered a large room near the dining area. It was not about picking partners or looking cool, but rather about free expression and joyful encounter.

The music ranged from new age to rock. Each individual allowed their bodies to move with the music as freely as their inhibitions would allow. Moving without the expectation of judgment felt freeing.

Then something unexpected happened. Without any outside instructions, people began randomly pairing up to dance with each other—sometimes mirroring movements, sometimes maintaining different styles, but always with a momentary sense of connection.

Without any verbal exchanges, I seemed to know when a dance with one person was over and then I danced comfortably alone until I sensed a connection with someone else. Each encounter felt nurturing—as if I had learned something about the other person as well as myself. There was a joyful sense of sharing and mutual creation without rules or conditions. It felt like a beautiful metaphor for the natural flow of relationships in an ideal world.

I had booked a professional massage late in the afternoon. The massage tables were on a top deck above the baths, and the combination of warm sun, cool breeze, and sea sounds took me again into trance. I could understand why some people gave up their "real life" to come and live at Esalen. My awareness drifted in and out as the massage took me to a level of emotional peace and physical relaxation that I had rarely experienced.

Esalen had captured me and I surrendered without a struggle. That evening, a bright full moon popped up over the coastal mountains and bathed the Esalen grounds in a magical light. I found a secluded spot where I did yoga postures and meditated late into the night.

I was still in trance when we drove home on Sunday. I was so "one with the universe" that the gas station pumps looked like beautiful works of art. No, I had not taken any drugs. The emotional high and sense of inner peace lasted for days after my return to Southern California.

My euphoria was a common phenomenon in growth groups and Esalen-type experiences. An artificial sense of closeness and connection is generated when interpersonal barriers are broken down rapidly. These feelings helped make encounter groups popular. For those without strong interpersonal connections in the real world, the "encounter group high" could be seductive to the point of addiction.

I was not addicted to encounter groups, but I was intoxicated by Esalen. The spectacular natural setting along with idealistic notions about people living up to their human potential led me to overlook some of the negative aspects of the community. As with any utopian effort, the reality falls short of the ideal. I was disappointed to discover that some of those in authority at Esalen were not as "fully developed" as I had hoped. The community suffered from some of the same "office politics" that are found in any organization. In addition, I eventually realized that some residents were more interested in experimentation with drugs and sex than in personal growth.

Nevertheless, Esalen and the ideals it represented are still magical to me.

-- Did you take any "magical mystery tours"—with or without the aid of chemicals?
-- What youthful ideals have you abandoned in the face of your experiences? To which ones do you still manage to cling?

Whiteboard Jungle Cruise

"Mr. Morgan, if you die in the earthquake do we still have to be quiet?" This is the question that Derrick blurts out during my opening day discussion of classroom safety and emergency procedures.

I pause and look at Derrick with a knowing grin. He is testing me. I respond with a slow, exaggerated cadence, "No Derrick, if I die in the earthquake you do not have to remain quiet." Sometimes it is important to let them win. My smile tells him that I appreciate his humor. I can tell that Derrick is going to be a fun student.

Perhaps I should clarify my choice of title. I am not Glenn Ford in a poverty devastated inner city classroom. My students are mostly white, middle-class suburbanites. They think they are poor if their parents don't buy them a car for their sixteenth birthday. Their story is not about overcoming the ravages of social injustice.

When I was a child, one of my favorite rides at Disneyland was the Jungle Cruise. I remember the air of adventure that I felt as I waited in line to board the riverboats. Part of me wanted to believe that I was in darkest Africa with a chance of losing an arm or a leg to a snapping crocodile or having our boat crushed by a charging hippo. The captain always managed to shoot the crocodiles and hippos just "in the nick of time" to save us. There was a surprise around every corner.

(The Disney ride has changed today since it is not politically correct to shoot endangered wildlife.)

This is the nature of my high school science classroom. Every day, usually when I least expected it, the kids surprised me. This is why I lost sleep the night before school opened—for over thirty-four years. It is fun to be the captain when most of the crew are volunteers who are well trained and rowing in the same direction. That is *not* the case in public high school. Each year I feared that my new crew would be filled with conscripts who have little motivation to even put their oars in the water—and might even delight in rowing in the wrong direction. Fear of mutiny always cost this captain a good night's sleep.

This opening day started as follows:

Directions clearly written on the whiteboard – check.
Handouts and materials ready – check.
Roll sheets and student schedules available – check.
My fly zipped up – check.

The first bell rings. Here we go. It's showtime.

I meet the students at the door and welcome them as they come in. Just before the tardy bell rings, in walks Amanda. Her makeup attempts to hide her insecurities, its thickness measured in millimeters. As she walks past me, I notice that she has no clothes on. Almost.

Amanda's blouse is so sheer that it is nearly invisible—completely revealing her black bra underneath. I didn't even make it to the bell before my first intervention. Not wanting to embarrass her, I ask her to step outside the room.

"Your clothing is not appropriate for school," I begin.

"It's the fashion!" she counters as she rolls her eyes in disgust. She wants me to know how out of it I am.

"It may be the fashion, but you can't wear that to school." I keep my voice calm to avoid escalation. I don't want to sound like her father.

"What's the big deal?" she continues. Actually, there are two big deals and they are very exposed. I don't share my thoughts or reveal the smile that wants to follow them. I need to get back to my class.

"I want you to go see the nurse. I will call and tell her that you are coming." I move toward the door to let her know that our discussion is over. Amanda says no more. Before she turns to walk toward the office, I think I notice moisture forming in the corners of her eyes. There is a lot more going on here than fashion choices.

As I walk across the back of the room, I survey the scene. The front three seats in every row are empty (They have ignored the first instruction on the board). The lab tables at the back of the room are crowded with loud talking students who act as if they are at a class reunion. They have all known each other for years, grouped into the same classes together. I am the outsider.

"Do not sit at lab tables!" I broadcast in my most authoritative voice.

"Sit at a desk and follow the instructions on the board." They move slowly, some groaning and others poking their friends as they relocate. The nonverbal message is not one of enthusiasm for learning.

The tardy bell rings as I call the nurse and ask her to talk with Amanda. I am frustrated because I like to start my classes right on time, especially on the first day.

I have just begun to introduce myself when the door opens and an electric wheelchair enters and begins to make its way across the back of the classroom. Harold, a young man with cerebral palsy, is trying to maneuver his vehicle through the overcrowded classroom, bumping into desks and lab tables as he goes. The class is enjoying the diversion. So much for setting the tone in my opening remarks.

Just when I think it might be safe to resume because Harold has settled into his parking spot, he shouts across the room in my direction, "My flaky aide didn't show up today." It is clear that Harold is no shrinking violet. I can already tell that he enjoys the class attention.

As I ponder how to respond to Harold's declaration, up pops another one of those surprises, this time a hand in the front row. "I can help Harold." My faith in humanity is restored. Michael will move next to Harold and help him get his notebook out of the backpack strapped to the back of his wheelchair.

Now, perhaps I can begin. I get the class's attention back and start to speak. Again, the door to the classroom opens. In comes a teacher with a frail looking, dark haired girl who seems to be hiding behind her. I move to greet them at the edge of the classroom.

"This is Christina," the teacher says, "she is going to be in your life science class this year."

I say "Hi Christina," and attempt to make eye contact with her. She will not look back at me, her head falling instead as she seems to focus on the floor.

"Christina is very *special*," says the teacher as she gives me a knowing wink. "She likes to sit in the back of the room by herself."

I guide Christina to a lab table in the rear of the class. When I turn around, the teacher is gone. That's it. That is the extent of the professional conversation I have about Christina, who obviously has some special needs. I am angry at the special ed teacher who has acted so unprofessionally, but I can't deal with it now.

I take a deep breath as I make my way back to the front of the room. Once again, I have to restore order. Once again, I begin to speak. Once again, the door opens. In walk three defiant looking sophomore boys. I'm hoping they have the wrong room. They don't. I take another deep breath.

"What happened?" I ask.

"We were talking with the principal." volunteers one of them, as if that sentence should be a reasonable justification for their tardiness. The other two are holding back a smile.

"Check their breath—I think they are drunk!" shouts Jake from the last row. I am afraid Jake might be right, but I'm not going down that road right now.

"Why were you talking with the principal?" I ask. I can see the wheels turning as they decide how far to take this.

"She stopped us because we were coming back late from lunch." They have decided not to push it on this first encounter with their new teacher.

"I'll talk with you at the end of class," I conclude our conversation. The three sit down.

Back to the front of the room. Restore order. Begin speaking. Harold shouts from his parking spot in the back corner, "I'm a commie."

Again, I am speechless.

"I look like Lenin and I am a commie," he continues.

185

This is going to be an E-ticket ride, I think. (If you are too young to understand this reference, Disneyland used to have separate ticket types for different categories of attractions. The fun rides—like the Matterhorn rollercoaster—required the more expensive "E" tickets.)

I decide I need to reign in Harold and begin to set the ground rules for the class. I explain to him that he needs to raise his hand and wait for recognition before speaking. Of course, in the middle of my sentence, his hand shoots up. It is not fully extended and sort of flails around because Harold has limited muscle control.

I don't take the bait, telling him that I will answer his question later because I need to begin class.

"Shall I make a puddle right here?" he asks—without being recognized. Score one for Harold. The class is laughing and I am smiling.

"If it is an emergency, take this pass and you may go," I say, trying to restore some authority. Harold starts bumping his way across the back of the room toward the door. He exchanges low volume retorts with several boys along the way. I think Harold has suggested that they perform unnatural acts on themselves, but I don't say anything. I meet Harold at the door with the pass and bend down to look him right in the eye.

"When you come back, I think it would be better if you sit right here by the door. Also, those kinds of comments are not appropriate for the classroom." We share a moment of face-to-face silence. It is amazing how powerful proximity can be.

"I understand," he says. I open the door for him and with a push of the control, he zooms out into the hallway.

Just as I again reach the front of the class, in walks Amanda. The nurse has given her an extra large T-shirt, which covers more than her whole outfit did before. She gives me a look of frustration as she sits, but I see a hint of relief as well. Once she got to school, I don't think she was very comfortable in the clothes she selected

Finally, I start my introduction and intended lesson plan. Even Harold manages to reenter the room and take his new position without disruption. There is no mutiny and I feel good about the day.

When I recite to other teachers and administrators the list of students I have in this class, their universal response was "Oh my God." Of my thirty-six students, twenty-five are boys. Most of them are on a first name basis with the assistant principal of discipline.

The three boys who were tardy all had parents who were absent or abusive and at various stages of drug or alcohol addiction. Later in the semester, the three were arrested for shoplifting at the nearby market on their lunch break. Ultimately they were all transferred to continuation school, but it took several months of "processing."

Even after they left, there were ten or twelve other boys vying for the title of "most obnoxious." Each of them had their own story. I learned some of them but could only guess at others. I realized early in my teaching career that I could not "save" every student in my classes. I looked for opportunities for impact where I could find them.

When I got to know Amanda, I discovered that she was new to the school. Her first-day fashion and makeup choices were the result of a bad guess about what would help her fit in.

Amanda quickly picked up the "beach casual" fashion style that predominated at our school. Her father was absent from her life, a common pattern I notice in girls who are flirtatious or excessive in their dress. She didn't stay mad at me after the first day. She thrived on the occasional attention and positive reinforcement that I was able to give her in class.

Harold was fun. He learned to judge when he could joke around with me and when it was time to relinquish the spotlight. He had a very bright mind and asked many great questions. He spoke with difficulty, slurring his words. He had learned to take the offensive when other students made fun of him by quickly making retorts that were often quite funny—though not quite appropriate for the classroom. More than one of his fellow students was offered the privilege of "wiping his ass" after they made a rude comment. (He actually did need assistance in the bathroom.)

Harold had been through several foster homes and would sometimes stay after class to talk about his life. He wanted to be a doctor—to find a cure for cerebral palsy. It helped when I explained the biological basis of his disease. Sometimes he felt that his condition was a punishment for something.

Harold transferred to another school before the year was out. During the transition, he was to have another surgery on the tendons in his hands, which were always rigidly tensed. I wished him well, told him I enjoyed his sense of humor, and praised his courage and perseverance.

As I suspected, Derrick turned out to be smart. I won his trust by treating him with respect and letting him know that dyslexia did not mean he was stupid. When I gave him extra time on tests and allowed him to complete some assignments orally, he earned an "A" in the class. I let him help me with lab set-ups and other tasks. He was never a behavior problem after he felt successful. I think his self-image changed when I suggested that he take college prep biology the next year.

When I tracked down Christina's special ed teacher, she told me that Christina had very limited abilities and had never been successful in a regular class before. She said that Christina's parents (who were both professionals) had insisted on placing her in my class against her recommendation. I couldn't believe it when the teacher said that it would be best if I *failed* Christina quickly to prove that she did not belong in regular classes.

For the first several weeks, Christina never spoke in my class, even to me. I discovered that if I explained the assignments carefully and gave her extra time, she could actually do quite well. I let her take her class assignments home and bring them back the next day.

Christina's parents were happy to work with her and I rewarded her efforts with good grades. You can't imagine how her face would light up when she got a paper back with an "A" or "B" grade on it. She became one of the hardest working students I have ever had, definitely slow but always steady. When she passed her first open note test, I let her take it home because she wanted to show her parents.

I felt like I had reached a real milestone when, for the first time, she left her seat in the back of the room, walked up to my desk, and asked a question about an assignment. I think I almost cried on the spot.

Christina earned a "B" for the semester and no student had ever deserved it more. I have more respect for that girl than for many of the gifted students I have had over the years.

At the beginning of the second semester, I received a call from Christina's father. We had spoken before when I called home to praise Christina for her hard work in my class. He told me that he had been transferred at work and the family was going to have to move to Texas right away. Then he said, "Mr. Morgan, I want to thank you from the bottom of my heart. You have changed Christina's life. Her behavior and her feelings about herself have been completely different since she found success in your class. We will always be grateful to you."

That is why I became a teacher.

-- Who was a positive influence in your life?
-- How has your life positively affected others?

Cows on Parade

My high school basketball coach was stereotypical of the post-war years of the '50s and early '60s. He brought a military attitude to preparation for battle on the hardwood. He emphasized discipline and sacrificing for the team. We started each practice with calisthenics and ended each practice running "four-liners" until we felt like throwing up. Drinking water during practice was for sissies.

Coach's hair was always military short. If you wanted to stay on the team, you followed his lead by keeping your hair "above the ears." We all wore ties on game day.

Sometime in the mid-'70s, I went back to my old high school to watch a basketball game. I knew my coach was still there, but I wasn't prepared for what I saw. His hair was nearly shoulder length, with big mutton chop sideburns. He had on a polyester shirt with a wide "disco" collar—and no tie. Most of his players had hair longer than his. I was stunned.

What I learned that night was the power of fads and peer pressure. My conservative coach was just changing with the times—unconsciously I am sure.

We have all seen fads come and go over the decades. They seem to wash in like seaweed on the beach, only to wash out with the next tide.

As a high school teacher, I had a front row seat for the style parade. One year the cool students would be in hippie-tie-die shirts, ragged jeans, and sandals. By the next September, following herd instincts I never comprehended,

191

the girls would show up wearing sequined blouses, tight designer jeans, and high heels! It was quite fascinating to watch.

I am a long way from being a slave to fashion. Yet I must admit to being seduced by the culture. I began my teaching career with short hair, wearing a coat and tie to class every day. In only a few years (after earning tenure) I am embarrassed to admit that I had a white man's afro and taught in caftan collarless shirts. When I confessed my fashion faux pas to my own children, they would not believe me—until I showed them the photos. That was a mistake.

Language is also faddish, especially in the young. When I was in high school, words like "boss," "cherry," or "bitchin" were common. When I began teaching, they had been replaced by "groovy," "right on," and "far out."

By the 1980s, hippy vocabulary was taboo on campus, replaced by a new dictionary of slang. "Killer" could be good or bad, as in "killer wave" or "killer test." "Bummers" were bad. Good things were "rad." The prefix "mega" meant extra, as in "mega-rad" or "mega-bummer."

Even after our culture embraced "do your own thing" liberation, we seem to like being part of the herd.

-- Which fashion or vocabulary fads (that you have observed or participated in) bring a smile to your face?

Bearly Walking

"The best-laid plans of mice and men often go awry"
-adapted from Robert Burns

This was the plan. Kasey and I would have some father-son bonding time during a short backpacking trip through the high country of Yosemite. We would establish a base camp below Half Dome and from there it would be a relatively easy ascent to the 8,842 foot summit. I would demonstrate my courage, strength, and wilderness skills to my son and he would have the lasting memory of the two of us conquering the mountain together.

That was the plan.

By the time we got off the bus at the Glacier Point trailhead, it was almost 11 a.m. The sun was bright and the air was already warm. In an effort to reduce the burden on my teenage son, I was carrying our tent, food, and cooking gear in addition to my clothes and sleeping bag. My backpack was heavy. Yet I was not concerned because I had done some conditioning walks at home and had a sturdy pair of leather hiking boots for support. We started out.

I expected a fairly level walk this first day because Glacier Point and our destination of Little Yosemite Valley were close to the same elevation. If I had studied the topographic map of the Panorama Trail more closely, however, I would have noticed that it was anything but level.

193

After a comfortable start, we began a series of steep switchbacks into the canyon created by Illilouette Creek. By the time we reached the footbridge that crossed the cascade, we had traveled two miles and dropped 1,200 feet in elevation. It was wonderful to sit by the beautiful rushing water—but after a brief rest, we had to climb out of the gorge on the other side of the Creek.

By now, the air was definitely hot and there were few trees along the trail. With each step, my pack got heavier. I was dripping sweat, my feet hurt, and I was puffing like a locomotive as I trudged up the trail to regain our elevation. I did not like the idea that Kasey could see me struggling. I knew he was getting frustrated with my slow pace and frequent stops for rest. In time he offered to carry some of the weight in my pack. I was embarrassed, but I didn't refuse his offer. I was worried that I had "bitten off more than I could chew" (to use one of my Dad's phrases).

By the time we finally reached Little Yosemite Valley, we had hiked almost six miles with 4,000 feet of elevation change and I was completely exhausted. My heart was pounding so hard I seriously thought I might have a heart attack right there on the spot. I lay down on the ground feeling lightheaded and too weak to move. My body was done.

It was close to an hour before I recovered enough strength to take off my boots. They had been good quality boots—when I had purchased them twenty years before. Now their once supple leather was dry and stiff. My feet had battled them throughout the hike—and had lost badly.

When I gingerly took off my socks, I saw that I had big blisters on my heels and my toes were completely black and blue. (A few days later, all of my toenails would fall off.) I applied some first aid to the blisters and reluctantly put my socks and boots back on. Although I was in pain, I decided I might actually live.

As we organized to cook dinner, a park ranger came by. He told us that a bear had disturbed the camp each of the past several nights. He warned us that the mother bear had cubs and had been very aggressive in her search for food. I knew that this news was unsettling for Kasey, and I tried not to let him see that I was also worried. I was very glad I had rented a "bear proof" food canister before we left the Valley.

As we later prepared to go to sleep, we made sure that anything aromatic (food, chapstick, toothpaste, etc.) was in the canister outside of our tent. Because of the Ranger's warning, my bear radar was turned on and I could not sleep. Every noise was magnified and grabbed my attention.

After what seemed like hours of semi-wakefulness, a commotion rose in the distance. Shouting people and banging pans broke the silence. Other backpackers were camped in the area, and the bear was systematically paying them a visit. Then it got quiet again.

Now I was wide-awake. A short time later, I heard another burst of sound that seemed a little closer. Then again, it got quiet. I strained to hear anything that would give me a clue as to the bear's movements.

I thought I heard a sound close by, a breaking twig perhaps. Suddenly, I felt the side of the tent pushed in next to my head and I heard what sounded like a sniff. My heart was pounding out of my chest.

"Kasey," I whispered, "I think the bear is here." I did my best not to sound panicky. Now we were both listening, breathing through our mouths to make as little noise as possible. We both heard rustling and scratching sounds that seemed to come from a few feet away on my side of the tent.

"Get the pans ready," I said as I fumbled to find the flashlight. I lifted up the window flap and shined the flashlight into the dark. There she was, a 300-pound black bear about three or four yards from my side of the tent.

"Kasey, she is going through our packs!" I said. Kasey leaned toward me to get a better look and just then, the bear noticed the light and turned to face us. Her eyes glowed bright red in the reflected light as she stared us down. I thought I was looking at the devil herself.

Then, without warning, she charged the tent.

I shrieked at the top of my lungs. I was hoping that Kasey would think I was still in control and trying to scare the bear away. In reality, I was completely terrified and my voice sounded like a woman screaming in a horror movie. Fortunately, Kasey was also yelling and may not have known the difference. We both rolled with our backs to the bear and waited for death.

Nothing happened. We stopped screaming and heard only silence. The tent was not crushed. The bear was not on top of us. We were not eaten. It had been like a bad nightmare and we had suddenly awakened. We heard no more from the bear—but neither one of us slept much.

The next morning, we examined the scene. Our packs had been rifled. My sunglasses case had a bear tooth indentation. There were "skid marks" where the bear had slid to a halt right at the edge of our tent. We could not believe it.

When I put on my "wooden" hiking boots, I realized that I could not go on to the summit of Half Dome. I was in too much pain and I was concerned about my ability get back down the mountain if I injured myself further. I dreaded the thought of disappointing Kasey, but I broke the news to him over breakfast.

I was surprised by his immediate response—he wanted to go on by himself. In fact, he was very determined. That put me in a dilemma. I was deeply worried about his safety, but I hated to be the one to keep him from attaining his goal.

I considered that this was one of the most heavily traveled trails in the world and he would be able to get help if he needed it. With great reluctance, I told him to go ahead without me.

I am so glad I did. Although I spent several nerve-racking hours waiting for his return, he successfully achieved his goal. From our camp, he had hiked the seven-mile round trip. He also conquered his fear of heights and negotiated the perilous cables that lead to the summit of Half Dome. It was a wonderful accomplishment.

Things had not gone as planned, but Kasey and I have memories that we will never forget.

-- When did your best-laid plans go awry—with memorable results?

Teach Your Children Well

You have had fifty years or more of life. So what wisdom would you pass on? Here is my list:

Humans are crazy. Our behavior rarely looks rational because our primary motivations are emotional and subconscious. Cut yourself and others some slack. Be understanding.

Humility is well deserved. We are all imperfect. We all fall short. Life satisfaction requires a balance between striving for improvement and self-acceptance. Be humble.

Live in the present. Regret for the past and worry about the future detract from the joy of life. Be mindful.

Everyone deserves compassion. We all have been hurt. We all have our fears. No matter the image we may project, inside we all need love and care. Be kind.

Giving is a key to happiness. In the final accounting, doing for others brings the deepest fulfillment. Be generous.

Gratitude is the best attitude. Each of us is better because of others generosity. Be appreciative.

The Golden Rule is golden. There is no better prescription for satisfying relationships, both personal and social.
Be considerate.

-- What life lessons do you want to pass along to your grandchildren (or other youth)?

Ask Not For Whom the Clock Ticks

If you are among the youngest Boomers (age fifty-two as I write this book in 2016), on average you have about 3 decades of life left (28 years for men, 31 for women). Thankfully, life expectancy continues to increase and our longevity as Boomers may improve upon the current data.

If you are among the oldest Boomers, you are turning seventy this year. Statistics say that on average you have about 14 more trips around the sun if you are male and perhaps 16 if you are female.

I don't know about you, but as an older Boomer, I am not happy about this. It doesn't feel like much time.

I clearly remember the joy I felt when the school year was over in elementary school. September to June seemed like an interminable length of time. Now the calendar year is half over before I start writing the correct date on my checks. The last decade of my life has flashed by like a Formula One car at the Indy 500. I barely had the chance to look at it before it was gone.

It may help to keep in mind that life expectancy is an average. It includes the people that overeat, smoke, and drive drunk. It includes the people who watch TV for more hours a day than they sleep. It includes the people whose main form of exercise is walking from the couch to the refrigerator.

I've always thought of myself as above average. I hold the attitude that my health habits will help me squeeze out a few extra years.

199

Whether we have three days, three years, or thirty years to live is unknown to us. Therefore, the important question is not "how long will I live," but simply "how will I live." Our challenge is to live the fullest, most satisfying, most fulfilling life possible, no matter the duration.

Life is uncertain. Eat dessert first. You may have seen this famous quote by Ernestine Ulmer on a poster or embroidered on a decorative pillow. It is one of my favorite sayings. To me, it means do not postpone your good. Think of the couple who spends their life dreaming of a tropical vacation in Hawaii, always waiting for the "right time" or to save "enough money." When they finally decide to travel, they may be too infirm to enjoy their dream. Or worse, one of them may be gone.

Carpe diem! (seize the day!) First written by the Roman poet Horace, the phrase was reborn in the movie *Dead Poets Society.* Teacher John Keating (Robin Williams) exhorts his students to "Carpe Diem! Seize the day, boys. Make your lives extraordinary!"

In the 1600s, Poet Robert Herrick expressed a similar sentiment:

> *Gather ye rosebuds while ye may.*
> *Old time is still a-flying;*
> *And this same flower that smiles today*
> *Tomorrow will be dying.*

Does this mean that our life should be a frantic dash to accumulate experiences? No. That would be an error at the other extreme. This is not the stage of life to burden ourselves with "to do" lists and "should" guilt. I've beaten myself up enough when I was younger.

Instead, I remind myself "I am enough. I have done enough." This attitude brings me peace of mind. My goal is to look for opportunities to live more fully while maintaining a balanced, stress-managed lifestyle. For me, how many years I live is not as important as how much living I do during my years.

For example, if I notice sunset colors in my late afternoon window, I stop what I am doing to go outside and enjoy nature's greatest show. If I am walking around my neighborhood, I walk a little slower to take in the old trees, new flowers, and ethereal clouds. If my granddaughter is visiting, I postpone my chores to focus fully on the delight in her laughter.

The new buzzword for this attitude in *mindfulness*. For me, Carpe Diem is not about how *much* you do, but how much appreciation and joy you can savor from *all* that you do.

-- What good in your life are you postponing? Why?
-- How do you keep yourself from living each day to the fullest?

You Know You're Old When...

...you hear snap, crackle, pop at the breakfast table—and you're not eating cereal.

...it takes two tries to get up from the couch.

...most names in your address book begin with Dr.

...you try to straighten out the wrinkles in your socks—and realize you aren't wearing any.

...the house catches fire and the first thing you grab is your Metamucil.

...you hear your favorite song in an elevator.

...you are on a first name basis with your pharmacist.

...your knees buckle and your belt won't.

...you have too much room in the house and not enough in the medicine cabinet.

...people call at 9 p.m. and ask, "Did I wake you?"

...you don't know a single song that wins a Grammy.

...you give up all your bad habits and still don't feel good.

...you would rather talk on the phone than text.

...you have a party and the neighbors don't notice.

You Know You're Old When...

...the twinkle in your eye is only a reflection off your bifocals.

...a sexy girl walks by and your pacemaker opens the garage door.

...going braless pulls all the wrinkles out of your face.

...you are warned to slow down by your doctor instead of the police.

...you consider going to the post office a busy day.

...you read the obituaries to check on your friends.

...you can live without sex but not your glasses.

...you can't remember what day it is and you don't care.

...you race to bring in your garbage cans before your neighbor.

...other drivers shake their head as they pass you.

...you think "hooking up" involves an RV.

...when a middle-aged guy calls you sir (or ma'am).

...five o'clock seems like a reasonable time to eat dinner.

...you're asleep, but others worry you're dead.

-- What makes you feel old?

Aging Staging

In 1969, Elizabeth Kubler-Ross published her groundbreaking book *On Death and Dying*. With acknowledgment of her influential work on the emotional responses to the experience of dying, I offer the following:

<u>On Age and Aging</u>

<u>Denial</u> – We all understand this one. The standard definition involves "imagining a preferred reality." You have undoubtedly noticed that I have developed this ability to a dangerously high level.

<u>Anger</u> – "How can this happen to me!" Whenever possible, this is accompanied by assigning blame. "This can't be *my* fault. Who is responsible for this!"

<u>Bargaining</u> – Negotiating with a higher power (or your own body) in exchange for a reformed lifestyle. "Stop this diarrhea and I will never eat chili again."

<u>Depression</u> – "With these health problems...," *or* "With these physical limitations...," *or* "With these aches and pains..., ...life is not worth living."

<u>Acceptance</u> – Embracing the disquieting future with a calm, positive attitude. "I may not be able to run or play competitive tennis anymore, but I can still hike and play pickleball!"

-- What stage are you in?

Life's Great Mysteries

In my nearly seven decades, I have figured out a lot of stuff. Here are some things that remain mysterious to me:

Who decided it is a fashion faux pas to wear socks with sandals? (My wife forbids Velcro shoes too.)

Why did fanny packs go from popular to taboo overnight? (I thought they were practical.)

Who thought ketchup packets were a good idea? (I never use them without getting ketchup on my fingers.)

Why do suburban white kids want to be "ghetto?"

Why is it hard to admit that I loved Barry Manilow?

When did humility go out of style?

Who decided that jeans would be the standard casual dress code for our generation? (They are bulky and heavy. Who needs thick denim unless you are a construction worker or ranch hand? Congrats to Levi's marketing department.)

Why can I remember commercial jingles from the '60s, but not what I had for lunch? Examples:

Brusha, brusha, brusha, with the new Ipana. (toothpaste)

Plop, plop, fizz, fizz, oh what a relief it is. (Alka Selzer)

Sometimes you feel like a nut.
Sometimes you don't.
Almond Joy's got nuts, Mounds don't.

You can hear the music in your head, can't you? How amazing that our mind can recreate the melodies all these decades later. It remains a scientific mystery.

To see how successful Madison Avenue has been at infiltrating our brains, fill in the following product names:

Melts in your mouth, not in your hand. _____

Please don't squeeze the _____.

Your in good hands with _____.

Ask any mermaid you happen to see,
What's the best tuna? _____ __ ___ ___.

Double your pleasure, double your fun
with _____, _____, _____ ___.

You'll wonder where the yellow went,
when you brush your teeth with _____.

Oh, I'd love to be an _____ _____ _____.

I know why I remember this next one. I used to sing it (pronoun modified) as I served food in the cafeteria line of the women's dorm when I was a freshman in college:
Feed her Doctor Ross dog food,
Do her a favor,
It's got more meat, and it's got more flavor.
It's got more meat to make her feel the way she should,
Doctor Ross dog food is doggone good. Woof!

(No mystery about why I didn't get many dates.)

_____

-- What makes you say "Are you kidding me?"
-- What other commercial jingles do you remember?

Mortality Sucks

There is at least one thing about which I am not in denial. I acknowledge death. In fact, I am financially, socially, and emotionally prepared for death.

Financially – Happily, all of our children are successful and self-sufficient. My wife and I enjoy giving to them and to our grandchildren, but we also feel free to use our resources to enjoy ourselves—to savor the fruits of our labor.

I live by the philosophy that you should support the organizations and causes that nourish you. I give to non-profits and charities that share my values and do good work in the world. I have updated my will and trust to reflect this philosophy. My children understand that they won't be able to retire on their inheritance.

Socially – One of the positives about death (now there is an odd statement) is that it motivates me to keep my relationships up to date. In my youth, it was reasonable to expect that everybody I cared about would be around the next day. Uncomfortable expressions of emotion could be safely postponed. That is no longer the case. The older I get, the more likely that someone I care about will be gone the next day (including myself!).

I strive to keep my relationships current. I especially try to express my love and appreciation to friends and family whenever I can. Back in the encounter group days of the '70s and '80s, we called it *taking care of unfinished business*. I want to leave as little unfinished business as possible.

Emotionally – I will be honest enough to admit to some fear of death. I do not like discomfort and pain. If that can be avoided, I think I can accept death. (Not that my acceptance will make a difference.)

The idea of not *being* (at least in this form) feels a little strange. Why did I worry so much about things that will ultimately mean nothing? Did it really matter whether I got an A- or B+ in that botony class? (If one of my grandchildren is reading this—yes it DOES matter!)

Everyone who saw me mess-up that speech, or heard me call them by the wrong name, (or noticed me wearing socks with sandals) will soon be dead! Why did I sweat the small stuff? (To demonstrate my personal growth, I have purposely included some imperfections in this writing ; -)

I don't need to expound on my spiritual beliefs here. (I was taught that it is not polite to discuss politics or religion with strangers.) Suffice to say that my belief system provides comfort without delusion. I do approach my nonexistence on this planet with regret because I have really enjoyed life. Nevertheless, as a part of the natural order, I can fully accept the inevitable.

I am not in denial about death. I accept death. I have prepared for death. My funeral arrangements have been made so that I will not be a burden to those that I love.

Now I can spend my precious time focused on savoring life.

-- What are you looking forward to at this stage of life?
-- Will you be financially, socially, and emotionally prepared to die when the time comes?

The Lasts

I am riding my bike around Yosemite Valley. The morning air is cool on my face and the sun is warm on my shoulders. I stop to admire the falls. The drought-reduced flow is even more beautiful than normal as the wispy veil of water shifts gracefully in the breeze. Surrounded by three thousand foot granite cliffs, I pass through open meadows and dense pine forests, occasionally paralleling the tranquil Merced River. For me, this is a peak experience. Nothing is more invigorating—or more spiritually satisfying.

As I shift gears on my aging hybrid bike, I wonder if I should replace it. It occurs to me that if I were to buy a new bike, it would certainly be my last. I smile at the thought. It reminds me of my last year of teaching.

During that year, I was nostalgically conscious as I taught each lesson. Last time I would demonstrate the rainbow that exists as white light. Last time I would explain DNA replication. Last time I would teach the pneumonic for the stages of mitosis. Last time I would tell this corny joke—and hear the students groan.

Aging can be another series of lasts. Last time to hike to Nevada Falls. Last time to sleep on the ground in a tent. Last time to float the river in a raft. Last time to ride a bike. Last time to ...

Perhaps the lesson of lasts is to *savor*. Savor each activity with deep appreciation. You never know if this time will be the last.

-- What "lasts" have you had? Which do you want to delay?

Remember When

Remember when airlines made you feel like a guest on a luxury cruise?

Remember when an attendant would greet you at a gas station, pump the gallons you wanted, and wash your windows without being asked?

Remember when you would call a business and a real person would answer the phone?

Remember when purchases came already assembled?

Remember when paying for a movie ticket meant you did not have to watch commercials at the theater?

How did we consumers get so disrespected in our modern world? *We* caused these changes by choosing price over quality. *We* caused these changes by continuing to patronize businesses that treated us poorly.

Airlines discovered that we were more interested in cheap tickets than in a quality travel experience. When two gas stations were on opposite corners, we chose the one that advertised the cheapest gas (even by a penny or two!), not the one that provided the best service. Businesses learned that if they replaced their customer service representatives with computer voices, they could lower their prices—and we would be *more* likely to buy their products because they were cheaper.

It's our own damn fault.

-- What do you miss about the "good old days?"

The Good Old Days?

Before we wax nostalgic about the "good old days," let's have a reality check:

Remember when smog was often so thick that it was hard to breathe? (You do if raised in the LA basin.)

Remember when our landfills were overflowing from mountains of unrecycled trash?

Remember when species were dying off due to the use of DDT and other pesticides?

Remember when toxic waste was dumped into pits and covered over—only to leach into water supplies?

Remember when cars had no seatbelts or airbags?

Remember when you had only seven television channels (three networks) to choose from? (If you were lucky.)

Remember searching for change to use a *pay* phone?

Remember when dog owners rarely cleaned up after their pets?

Remember when you had to figure out how to fold up a paper map?

Remember when there was no weather radar? (You had to stick your hand out to check if it was raining.)

Remember when jokes about race, ethnicity, gender, or sexual orientation were socially acceptable?

I don't embrace all of the changes we have seen. For example, texting is sometimes convenient, but it is no replacement for genuine conversation. And who wants their every physical move tracked by GPS and their every phone call and Internet search tracked by...who knows?

211

On the other hand, how cool is it to "Facetime" my grandson after he hits a home run during his little league game? How convenient to have a world of information accessible at the touch of a "Google" button? How marvelous will it be when self-driving cars bring automotive injuries and deaths to near zero. We have watched the evolution of technology beyond anything we could have dreamed as children.

Nonetheless, we still have problems to solve. People continue to kill each other in the name of religion. Civil war atrocities create thousands of refugees. Nations fight over resources like water, oil, and territory. Humans degrade the natural world and alter the climate in the pursuit of wealth.

If you watch the 24/7 cable news networks, you might start to believe that we are all doomed to die at the hands of terrorists or unprecedented weather events. When I get together with friends, it is easy to slip into a "What is wrong with the world?" conversation. But don't give up on the world. The fact is, *in most areas of human welfare we are making remarkable progress:*

Consider human violence.

The worldwide rate of death from war has gone down from 300/100,000 people during WWII; to 30 during the Korean War; to the low teens during the Vietnam War; to single digits at the end of the 20th century; to less than 1/100,000 people in the twenty-first century. Even if you count terrorism, humans are less likely to die in war today *than at any time in human history.*

The decline in war violence is even more dramatic if you take a longer view. For example, in Europe alone there was an average of two new interstate conflicts *per year* since the 1400s. There have been no interstate wars in Europe since 1945 (unless you count a brief incursion of the Soviet Union into Hungary in 1956).

The average number of international wars fought every year has declined from over six in the 1950s to less than one in the 2000s. From the 1990s, the deadliest conflicts (those that killed over 1000 people per year) have declined by more than half.

Battle deaths have also declined. In 1950, the annual rate of war dead was approximately 240 per million of the world's population. By 2007, it was less than 10 per million. To repeat, statistics tell us we are living in the most peaceful age in human history.

War is responsible for only one out of every ten violent deaths. The majority of the rest are the result of homicides. There has been a dramatic decline in murder rates over the centuries. Europe provides the most reliable statistics. In the 13th century, homicide accounted for between 40 and 80 deaths per 100,000 Europeans. By the end of the 20th century, rates had dropped to about 2 per 100,000.

The global homicide rate today is about 8 deaths per 100,000. The U.S. rate today is 4 per 100,000, down from a peak of 10 in 1980. Overall, violent crimes have declined in the U.S. from a peak of 758/100,000 in early 1991 to 387/100,000 in 2012—nearly a 50% decline.

Despite the horrific tragedies that have too frequently been in the headlines, the past 25 years have seen a dramatic *drop* in violent crimes on school campuses. In 1993, there were 42 student homicides per 100,000 students in the U.S. After years of steady decline, that number was 4 per 100,000 in 2010.

To highlight another form of violence, between 1973 and 2008, the incidence of rape in the U.S. has declined over 80%.

(Note: Because writing a scholarly work has not been my goal, I have not included references for my statistics. Steven Pinker has taken a comprehensive look at the decline in violence over human history in his book *The Better Angels of Our Nature*. I recommend it to any of you that want a thorough examination of the data.)

Many Americans list terrorism as their number one fear. Yet we are more likely to die from a lightning strike, a deer encounter, a bee sting, or our pajamas catching on fire, than at the hands of a terrorist.

How many more lives could have been saved if we had taken some of the 1 trillion dollars spent on homeland security since 9/11 and used it for lightening rods, dear fencing, EpiPens, or pajama safety education?

Of course, I am being humorous (sort of). But would the world be a safer place if we had used some of the 4 trillion dollars spent on the Afghanistan and Iraq wars to educate young Islamic minds instead of killing their bodies? Could we spend our national treasure more wisely if we didn't let fear overcome rationality? Can we begin to replace revenge with higher motives that accelerate our progress to a safer and more peaceful world?

(I guess this Boomer still believes in '60s idealism.)

Consider health and longevity.

According to the World Health Organization, between 1990 and 2013, mortality rates for children under five declined worldwide by nearly 50%, largely due to improved nutrition and vaccination programs. Polio has been 99% eradicated from the face of the earth (just a couple small pockets still exist in Pakistan and Afghanistan). It will soon join Smallpox on the list of completely eradicated diseases. Distribution of mosquito nets and insect repellents, draining standing water, and spraying of insecticides has reduced the worldwide rates of malaria by 37% between 2000 and 2015. The spread of HIV has been reversed with 2.1 million new cases in 2013, down from 3.4 million in 2001.

In 1990, 24% of the world's population did not have access to safe drinking water. By 2010, that figure had dropped to 11%.

Average life expectancy around the world has gone from 47 years in 1950 to 70 years in 2011.

Extreme poverty ($1.25/day) has dropped from 40% of the world's population in 1981 to 14% in 2010.

Consider political oppression.

There were only a handful of democracies around the globe following World War II. Although there remain notable dictatorships and authoritarian governments, over 60% of all countries are now democracies.

Nearly all countries of the world (193) are members of the United Nations, declaring themselves to be "peace-loving states."

Consider our natural environment.

Sixteen thousand species are listed as declining, threatened, or endangered. Climate change is adding to this number. This is beyond tragic—because extinction is forever.

On the positive side, the number of protected habitats around the world has grown from 10,000 in 1970 to over 100,000 today. Nations of the world have committed to extend protection to over 17% of all terrestrial habitats by 2020.

The cost of wind and solar energy is coming down so rapidly that it is no longer unrealistic to talk about a world completely powered by renewable energy. In 2015, 195 nations signed the Paris climate change accord, committing to a reduction in greenhouse gas emissions.

Ozone depletion in the atmosphere that reached crisis levels in the 1980s can serve as a model of environmental stewardship. In 1987, every United Nation's country signed the agreement to phase out the use of CFC's—chemicals that were destroying the ozone layer. Within 20 years, ozone depletion was reversed, with scientists estimating a return to 1980 levels by 2050.

The reduction of greenhouse gasses through the Paris Accord will be more challenging, but no less achievable.

Because of differences in personality and values, some people seem to enjoy focusing on the negative "ain't it awful" prospective. But if you want to know the *actual* state of the world, look at the *trend* lines, not the headlines. There is a great deal to inspire hope for humanity and our world.

We Changed the World (Didn't We?)

I like being a Boomer. It makes me feel special. After all, we are responsible for all the wonderful trends in the world, right? Our collective voices helped end an unjust war and stop the Draft. We began the environmental movement. Perhaps most importantly, we catalyzed dramatic progress in human rights and social justice.

We changed the world, didn't we?

We rejected the status quo—wearing clothes that advertised our differences from our parents and growing our hair as a sign of solidarity with each other. We turned folk music into protest rock to spread our message of peace and liberation. We redefined personal freedoms to include sex, drugs, (and rock and roll).

We transformed the culture, didn't we?

We were more informed, more socially conscious, more energized than any of those who came before or after us. No generation since has mounted a serious political or social protest. (Occupy Wall Street and Black Lives Matter were anemic attempts by comparison.) We believed in personal growth and transformation—whether through drugs, meditation, personal therapy, EST, or encounter groups.

That is how we became so evolved, right?

We are special, right?

It is easy to get all puffed-up about our generation. (No wonder we irritate the hell out of non-Boomers.)

What if it was not we who changed the world, but an evolving world that changed us? What if we were the *product* of change, rather than the *instigators* of change? Consider three examples:

1)   We commonly think that we invented *real* rock and roll as a vehicle to express our protest of the status quo — combining the socially conscious lyrics of folk music with the driving beat of rhythm and blues. But some have suggested that the rapid rise of rock and roll was less dependent on our evolving consciousness and more dependent on new technology like electric guitars and amplification.

And then along came the transistor. For the first time, adolescents with transistor radios did not have to sit in the living room and listen to the music of their parents. Music could evolve on separate tracks. Older listeners could keep their Frank Sinatra and Patti Page while their teenage children could listen to the Beatles and Rolling Stones.

2)   Perhaps it was not social rebellion as much as sophisticated marketing that moved rock and roll into the center of popular culture. In order to attract our bulging demographic (that advertisers coveted), radio stations dedicated to adolescent tastes emerged. Television programs like American Bandstand and Soul Train sought the same audience. Such programs not only sold records, they sold clothing, cosmetics, movies and more. Profits soared as Madison Avenue shaped our taste and taught us what to buy in order to stay socially acceptable to our peers.

Of course, our tastes had to be different than our parents. Our adolescent need for separation was deftly used to create style trends that sold merchandise.

3)   Wars are always protested by some. But the technology of global satellite relays of television signals may have multiplied the number of people who cared about Vietnam. For the first time, most homes in the country watched the daily horrors of war in their living rooms each evening— discussing the pros and cons of our national policies at the dinner table. At a naturally rebellious stage of life, we Boomers were quick to question our overseas involvement.

I also have to wonder if the energy of our protests would have been as great without the personal fear of being drafted. Were we more conscious, more noble than today's youth? Would we have rallied by the tens of thousands against an unjustified war if we and our friends were not being sent to the slaughter involuntarily? Would the wars in Afghanistan and Iraq have been possible if the Draft still put all of our nation's young people potentially in harm's way?

And just who is this "we" anyway?

Although many of us were sympathetic, few of the 75 million of us joined war protests in civil disobedience. Even fewer of us got on the buses to Alabama or Mississippi to fight for racial justice. It was a relative handful of Boomers (and many born before) who did the real work. If you were among that handful, you have my respect.

The rest of us Boomers should remain justifiably humble. We were in the right place at the right time—and went along for the cultural ride. We were not born unique. We *became* unique in response to evolving technology and social forces.

Still, we are Boomers. We are no longer rebellious youth, but we continue to support positive change. We can be proud of that.

Epilogue 2

In the introduction, I said:

I am writing this book because I enjoy writing. That has turned out to be an understatement. I have learned so much about my body—what is happening as I age and what I might expect in the future. Organizing the information presented here has helped my understanding.

I am writing this book because I like to reflect. Writing this book has transported me back in time. While I do not live in the past, I do like to visit occasionally. Some people, events, emotions, and experiences are worthy of a second look. Reflection has deepened my gratitude.

I am writing this book because I want to help others. My hope is that you found a few tidbits of information in this book to be helpful. I have been motivated by the thought that perhaps one person will be saved because their memory of stroke effects, heart attack symptoms, or cancer warning signs has been refreshed. If my admonition to get to a doctor when our body doesn't *feel right, look right, or work right* accelerates one Boomer's treatment intervention, I have succeeded.

Thanks for your support. I will appreciate your feedback if you want to email me (rwaynemorgan@comcast.net).

May we Boomers be the healthiest and happiest old farts that the planet has ever known.

All good wishes,
Wayne

Addendum: Hidden Treasures

I have shared my memories and musings with the goal of triggering some of your own. I know for me, a smell, a word, or a visual image can take me to places unvisited in decades. The brain is an astounding repository of memories—easily accessed with the proper stimulation.

The following items are not for casual reading. They expand upon the suggestions presented at the end of some of the previous essays of Section II. Take them one at a time. Allow the prompt to stimulate a memory. Enjoy it. Savor it. Follow the connections to other memories that may arise. This process could take you weeks to months if you want it to.

If you have ever thought about writing a memoir, this process could be a good starting point. Write about the people, events, and feelings that come to mind when you consider each of the following prompts (in addition to those in the previous essays.) You will be well on your way to telling your life's story.

Have fun!

---

1. What is your earliest memory?
2. What is your favorite memory of your parents?
3. What was your favorite toy as a child?
4. What is your first memory of school?
5. Who was your favorite elementary teacher?
6. Who was your favorite high school teacher?
7. When were you embarrassed at school?

8. When did you have a good laugh at school?
9. What did you like to play when you were alone?
10. What did you like to play with others?
11. What is the first house you remember?
12. What is a happy childhood memory?
13. What is a sad childhood memory?
14. When did you play a prank on someone?
15. What childhood event impacted your life?
16. Where did you go for summer vacations as a child?
17. What camp or school trip was memorable?
18. What was your favorite extracurricular activity?
19. What did you learn about yourself in high school?
20. Who gave you your first kiss?
21. What is your best teen memory with your friends?
22. What was your hometown like?
23. What was your first job?
24. What conversation had an impact on your life?
25. What song brings back memories for you?
26. Who do you wish you could see again?
27. What was the greatest challenge in your life?
28. What family heirloom do you still have?
29. What role has religion played in your life?
30. What events left scars (physical or psychological)?
31. What three people influenced you the most?
32. What are you passionate about?
33. What contest or competition did you participate in?
34. What was the first book that sticks in your mind?
35. What is your favorite holiday memory?
36. Who was the lost love of your life?
37. What was your favorite job or job project?
38. What regrets do you have?
39. When in life have you felt most loved?
40. What time in your life would you like to relive?

What is the first memory that comes to mind when you read the following words?

Recess
Pet
Surprise
Church (Temple)
Dance
Crush
Car
Date
Party
Car Bench Seat
Graduation
Wedding
Relative
Tradition

The portion of the brain involved in smell (olfactory bulb) is located near the areas responsible for memories (hippocampus and amygdala). Scents can thus trigger strong recollections. What memories are brought to mind when you imagine the following smells?

freshly mowed grass
new car
roasting turkey
hot radiator
dirty diaper
baking bread
cheap perfume
frying bacon
pine needles
sunscreen
roses

Index

Also by R. Wayne Morgan

My Favorite Wisdom:
   Notes to My Grandchildren about Life and Living

Sure, I Can Do That:
   A Twentieth Century American Memoir

The Fermata Chronicle:
   A Novella of the Next Age

The first is available in paperback. All three are available as eBooks. Just search on your favorite bookseller's website for R. Wayne Morgan.

Feel free to send suggestions, comments, or questions to:
rwaynemorgan@comcast.net

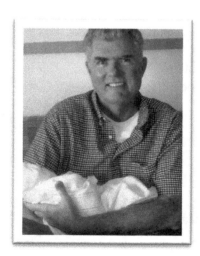

Author with Grandson